# CANINE EPILEPSY JOURNAL

*Keep a Diary of Your Dog's Seizures, Medications, Triggers*

*& Side Effects*

Medjournal Essentials

This Journal Belongs To: ................................................................

Dog's Name: ................................................................

## Vet Contact Information

Name: ................................................................

Practice Name: ................................................................

Telephone: ................................................................

Address: ................................................................

................................................................

................................................................

## Out of Hours Vet

Name: ................................................................

Practice Name: ................................................................

Telephone: ................................................................

Address: ................................................................

................................................................

................................................................

# CONTENTS

# Canine Epilepsy

KEEPING A SEIZURE LOG

❦

As the owner of a dog with epilepsy you face many challenges, one of which is keeping track of seizures, medications and side effects. This journal will help you keep that information together in one place. The records you keep will help you and your vet to reach decisions about treatment and help you see if treatments are effective. This journal is easy to use, and you can bring it to consultations with your vet.

## Why Is It Important to Keep a Seizure Log?

There are several important reasons for keeping a seizure log – to aid in diagnosis, to help your vet make decisions about treatment, and to help you spot warnings, patterns and triggers.

### *Diagnosis & Treatment Decisions*

Writing down what happens before, during and after a seizure can help your vet identify the type of seizures that your dog is having. This is important to know when prescribing medications. Keeping a record also helps you and your vet decide whether medications are effective or need changing. If seizures get better, stay the same, or get worse after a medication change everyone needs to know. A log will also help you track side effects your dog may be experiencing. Sometimes side effects settle down after a period of time, but sometimes they indicate a change in dose or medication is needed. All the information you gather helps you and your vet make informed decisions about treatment.

### *Patterns & Triggers*

Noting the time, where your dog was and what was going on prior to a seizure may help you spot patterns and identify potential triggers. Some common triggers are listed on the seizure record pages as tick box options, and there are spaces to record your own. There is also a notes section for your own observations and thoughts. Identifying triggers could help you find changes that may help (for example avoiding certain foods, stressful events or certain kinds of exercise). Keeping records will also help you see if the changes you introduce are making a difference.

# Using the Seizure Journal

*Seizure Calendar*

This journal has a calendar on which you can quickly record the number of seizures on any given day and easily spot frequency over days, weeks and months. You can see how many days have passed between events, or any patterns. More information on using the calendar and an example is included at the beginning of the calendar section.

*Medications*

Each medication that your dog is prescribed has its own page in which you can record the dosage and frequency, record changes and note any side effects.

*Questions to Ask Your Vet*

It can be difficult to remember everything you wanted to ask when you are in the consulting room, use this section to note down questions you have for your vet and bring it along with you.

*Seizure Log*

The log pages are written without using medical terms so that family members, dog sitters or kennels can update the log if needed. Only fill in the information sections that you need, skip any that are not relevant.

# One Last Thing

We are always looking to improve, and regularly review our journals to make sure they are meeting your needs. If you have a suggestion for something we can add to future revisions, want to let us know about something we do well, or something we could do better, please get in touch. We read every suggestion we receive and always appreciate your feedback.

Contact us on: customersupport@medjournalessentials.com

# Calendar

⚭

# Using the Seizure Calendar

Use the calendar to record the number of seizures that have happened on any given day. Fill in the year at the top and the current month on the left-hand side (or previous months if you wish to track historical data). If your dog only has one type of seizure, write the number in for that day. If your dog has several types of seizure, you can give each one a code (a chart is provided below) write the code followed by the number of seizures each day. Alternatively, you can write down the page number on which you have recorded seizures. If there has been a change in medication, or other changes such as a stay in kennels or change in diet, you can shade in the relevant days, weeks or months with a coloured pencil. This allows you to see if the changes have had an effect. A key is included below.

| Month | 1 | 2 | 3 | 4 | 5 | 6 |
|-------|-----|---|---|------|---|---|
| Jan   | F1<br>T2 |   |   | P.<br>32 |   |   |

| Seizure Type | Code |
|--------------|------|
|              |      |
|              |      |
|              |      |
|              |      |
|              |      |

| Colour | Medication / Other Change |
|--------|---------------------------|
|        |                           |
|        |                           |
|        |                           |
|        |                           |
|        |                           |
|        |                           |
|        |                           |
|        |                           |

# Seizure Calendar

Year: _____

| Month | 1 | 2 | 3 | 4 | 5 | 6 | 7 | 8 | 9 | 10 | 11 | 12 | 13 | 14 | 15 | 16 | 17 | 18 | 19 | 20 | 21 | 22 | 23 | 24 | 25 | 26 | 27 | 28 | 29 | 30 | 31 |
|-------|---|---|---|---|---|---|---|---|---|----|----|----|----|----|----|----|----|----|----|----|----|----|----|----|----|----|----|----|----|----|----|
|       |   |   |   |   |   |   |   |   |   |    |    |    |    |    |    |    |    |    |    |    |    |    |    |    |    |    |    |    |    |    |    |
|       |   |   |   |   |   |   |   |   |   |    |    |    |    |    |    |    |    |    |    |    |    |    |    |    |    |    |    |    |    |    |    |
|       |   |   |   |   |   |   |   |   |   |    |    |    |    |    |    |    |    |    |    |    |    |    |    |    |    |    |    |    |    |    |    |
|       |   |   |   |   |   |   |   |   |   |    |    |    |    |    |    |    |    |    |    |    |    |    |    |    |    |    |    |    |    |    |    |
|       |   |   |   |   |   |   |   |   |   |    |    |    |    |    |    |    |    |    |    |    |    |    |    |    |    |    |    |    |    |    |    |
|       |   |   |   |   |   |   |   |   |   |    |    |    |    |    |    |    |    |    |    |    |    |    |    |    |    |    |    |    |    |    |    |
|       |   |   |   |   |   |   |   |   |   |    |    |    |    |    |    |    |    |    |    |    |    |    |    |    |    |    |    |    |    |    |    |
|       |   |   |   |   |   |   |   |   |   |    |    |    |    |    |    |    |    |    |    |    |    |    |    |    |    |    |    |    |    |    |    |
|       |   |   |   |   |   |   |   |   |   |    |    |    |    |    |    |    |    |    |    |    |    |    |    |    |    |    |    |    |    |    |    |
|       |   |   |   |   |   |   |   |   |   |    |    |    |    |    |    |    |    |    |    |    |    |    |    |    |    |    |    |    |    |    |    |
|       |   |   |   |   |   |   |   |   |   |    |    |    |    |    |    |    |    |    |    |    |    |    |    |    |    |    |    |    |    |    |    |
|       |   |   |   |   |   |   |   |   |   |    |    |    |    |    |    |    |    |    |    |    |    |    |    |    |    |    |    |    |    |    |    |

# *Seizure Calendar*

Year: _____

| Month | 1 | 2 | 3 | 4 | 5 | 6 | 7 | 8 | 9 | 10 | 11 | 12 | 13 | 14 | 15 | 16 | 17 | 18 | 19 | 20 | 21 | 22 | 23 | 24 | 25 | 26 | 27 | 28 | 29 | 30 | 31 |
|---|---|---|---|---|---|---|---|---|---|---|---|---|---|---|---|---|---|---|---|---|---|---|---|---|---|---|---|---|---|---|---|
| | | | | | | | | | | | | | | | | | | | | | | | | | | | | | | | |
| | | | | | | | | | | | | | | | | | | | | | | | | | | | | | | | |
| | | | | | | | | | | | | | | | | | | | | | | | | | | | | | | | |
| | | | | | | | | | | | | | | | | | | | | | | | | | | | | | | | |
| | | | | | | | | | | | | | | | | | | | | | | | | | | | | | | | |
| | | | | | | | | | | | | | | | | | | | | | | | | | | | | | | | |
| | | | | | | | | | | | | | | | | | | | | | | | | | | | | | | | |
| | | | | | | | | | | | | | | | | | | | | | | | | | | | | | | | |
| | | | | | | | | | | | | | | | | | | | | | | | | | | | | | | | |
| | | | | | | | | | | | | | | | | | | | | | | | | | | | | | | | |
| | | | | | | | | | | | | | | | | | | | | | | | | | | | | | | | |
| | | | | | | | | | | | | | | | | | | | | | | | | | | | | | | | |

# *Seizure Calendar*

Year: _____

| Month | 1 | 2 | 3 | 4 | 5 | 6 | 7 | 8 | 9 | 10 | 11 | 12 | 13 | 14 | 15 | 16 | 17 | 18 | 19 | 20 | 21 | 22 | 23 | 24 | 25 | 26 | 27 | 28 | 29 | 30 | 31 |
|---|---|---|---|---|---|---|---|---|---|---|---|---|---|---|---|---|---|---|---|---|---|---|---|---|---|---|---|---|---|---|---|
| | | | | | | | | | | | | | | | | | | | | | | | | | | | | | | | |
| | | | | | | | | | | | | | | | | | | | | | | | | | | | | | | | |
| | | | | | | | | | | | | | | | | | | | | | | | | | | | | | | | |
| | | | | | | | | | | | | | | | | | | | | | | | | | | | | | | | |
| | | | | | | | | | | | | | | | | | | | | | | | | | | | | | | | |
| | | | | | | | | | | | | | | | | | | | | | | | | | | | | | | | |
| | | | | | | | | | | | | | | | | | | | | | | | | | | | | | | | |
| | | | | | | | | | | | | | | | | | | | | | | | | | | | | | | | |
| | | | | | | | | | | | | | | | | | | | | | | | | | | | | | | | |
| | | | | | | | | | | | | | | | | | | | | | | | | | | | | | | | |
| | | | | | | | | | | | | | | | | | | | | | | | | | | | | | | | |
| | | | | | | | | | | | | | | | | | | | | | | | | | | | | | | | |

# *Seizure Calendar*

Year: _____

| Month | 1 | 2 | 3 | 4 | 5 | 6 | 7 | 8 | 9 | 10 | 11 | 12 | 13 | 14 | 15 | 16 | 17 | 18 | 19 | 20 | 21 | 22 | 23 | 24 | 25 | 26 | 27 | 28 | 29 | 30 | 31 |
|---|---|---|---|---|---|---|---|---|---|---|---|---|---|---|---|---|---|---|---|---|---|---|---|---|---|---|---|---|---|---|---|
| | | | | | | | | | | | | | | | | | | | | | | | | | | | | | | | |
| | | | | | | | | | | | | | | | | | | | | | | | | | | | | | | | |
| | | | | | | | | | | | | | | | | | | | | | | | | | | | | | | | |
| | | | | | | | | | | | | | | | | | | | | | | | | | | | | | | | |
| | | | | | | | | | | | | | | | | | | | | | | | | | | | | | | | |
| | | | | | | | | | | | | | | | | | | | | | | | | | | | | | | | |
| | | | | | | | | | | | | | | | | | | | | | | | | | | | | | | | |
| | | | | | | | | | | | | | | | | | | | | | | | | | | | | | | | |
| | | | | | | | | | | | | | | | | | | | | | | | | | | | | | | | |
| | | | | | | | | | | | | | | | | | | | | | | | | | | | | | | | |
| | | | | | | | | | | | | | | | | | | | | | | | | | | | | | | | |
| | | | | | | | | | | | | | | | | | | | | | | | | | | | | | | | |

# Medication History

❧

# *Medication History*

| Medication & Dose | Date Started | Reason for Starting |
|---|---|---|
| | | |
| | Date Stopped | Reason for Stopping |
| | | |

## Changes

| Date | New Dose | Reason for Change |
|---|---|---|
| | | |
| | | |
| | | |
| | | |
| | | |

| Date | Side Effects / Notes |
|---|---|
| | |
| | |
| | |
| | |
| | |
| | |
| | |

# *Medication History*

| Medication & Dose | Date Started | Reason for Starting |
|---|---|---|
| | | |
| | Date Stopped | Reason for Stopping |
| | | |

## Changes

| Date | New Dose | Reason for Change |
|---|---|---|
| | | |
| | | |
| | | |
| | | |
| | | |

| Date | Side Effects / Notes |
|---|---|
| | |
| | |
| | |
| | |
| | |
| | |
| | |

# Medication History

| Medication & Dose | Date Started | Reason for Starting |
|---|---|---|
|  |  |  |
|  | Date Stopped | Reason for Stopping |
|  |  |  |

## Changes

| Date | New Dose | Reason for Change |
|---|---|---|
|  |  |  |
|  |  |  |
|  |  |  |
|  |  |  |
|  |  |  |

| Date | Side Effects / Notes |
|---|---|
|  |  |
|  |  |
|  |  |
|  |  |
|  |  |
|  |  |
|  |  |
|  |  |

# Medication History

| Medication & Dose | Date Started | Reason for Starting |
|---|---|---|
| | Date Stopped | Reason for Stopping |
| | | |

## Changes

| Date | New Dose | Reason for Change |
|---|---|---|
| | | |
| | | |
| | | |
| | | |
| | | |

| Date | Side Effects / Notes |
|---|---|
| | |
| | |
| | |
| | |
| | |
| | |
| | |

# *Medication History*

| Medication & Dose | Date Started | Reason for Starting |
|---|---|---|
| | | |
| | Date Stopped | Reason for Stopping |
| | | |

## Changes

| Date | New Dose | Reason for Change |
|---|---|---|
| | | |
| | | |
| | | |
| | | |
| | | |

| Date | Side Effects / Notes |
|---|---|
| | |
| | |
| | |
| | |
| | |
| | |
| | |
| | |

# *Medication History*

| Medication & Dose | Date Started | Reason for Starting |
|---|---|---|
| | | |
| | Date Stopped | Reason for Stopping |
| | | |

## Changes

| Date | New Dose | Reason for Change |
|---|---|---|
| | | |
| | | |
| | | |
| | | |
| | | |

| Date | Side Effects / Notes |
|---|---|
| | |
| | |
| | |
| | |
| | |
| | |
| | |
| | |

# *Medication History*

| Medication & Dose | Date Started | Reason for Starting |
|---|---|---|
| | | |
| | **Date Stopped** | **Reason for Stopping** |
| | | |

## Changes

| Date | New Dose | Reason for Change |
|---|---|---|
| | | |
| | | |
| | | |
| | | |
| | | |

| Date | Side Effects / Notes |
|---|---|
| | |
| | |
| | |
| | |
| | |
| | |
| | |
| | |

# *Medication History*

| Medication & Dose | Date Started | Reason for Starting |
|---|---|---|
|  |  |  |
|  | Date Stopped | Reason for Stopping |
|  |  |  |

## Changes

| Date | New Dose | Reason for Change |
|---|---|---|
|  |  |  |
|  |  |  |
|  |  |  |
|  |  |  |
|  |  |  |

| Date | Side Effects / Notes |
|---|---|
|  |  |
|  |  |
|  |  |
|  |  |
|  |  |
|  |  |
|  |  |

# *Medication History*

| Medication & Dose | Date Started | Reason for Starting |
|---|---|---|
| | | |
| | Date Stopped | Reason for Stopping |
| | | |

## Changes

| Date | New Dose | Reason for Change |
|---|---|---|
| | | |
| | | |
| | | |
| | | |
| | | |

| Date | Side Effects / Notes |
|---|---|
| | |
| | |
| | |
| | |
| | |
| | |
| | |
| | |

# *Medication History*

| Medication & Dose | Date Started | Reason for Starting |
|---|---|---|
| | | |
| | Date Stopped | Reason for Stopping |
| | | |

## Changes

| Date | New Dose | Reason for Change |
|---|---|---|
| | | |
| | | |
| | | |
| | | |
| | | |

| Date | Side Effects / Notes |
|---|---|
| | |
| | |
| | |
| | |
| | |
| | |
| | |
| | |

## Medication History

| Medication & Dose | Date Started | Reason for Starting |
|---|---|---|
|  |  |  |
|  | Date Stopped | Reason for Stopping |
|  |  |  |

## Changes

| Date | New Dose | Reason for Change |
|---|---|---|
|  |  |  |
|  |  |  |
|  |  |  |
|  |  |  |
|  |  |  |

| Date | Side Effects / Notes |
|---|---|
|  |  |
|  |  |
|  |  |
|  |  |
|  |  |
|  |  |
|  |  |
|  |  |

# Questions to Ask Your Vet

൭ൈ

# *Questions to Ask Your Vet*

## Questions to Ask Your Vet

# Questions to Ask Your Vet

# Seizure Log

☙❧

# Seizure Log

Date: _____ Time: _____ Duration: _____

Location: _____

Seizure Type: _____

If this was a cluster how many seizures? _____

Was your dog: Asleep ☐  Awake ☐  Waking from sleep ☐

What happened during the seizure? _____

_____

_____

_____

What was happening around the time the seizure occurred?

_____

_____

_____

Was there an Aura or warning? Yes ☐  No ☐  Describe: _____

_____

_____

Rescue medication if given: _____

Taken to vet? Yes ☐  No ☐  Detail: _____

How long did your dog take to recover? _____

Notes: _____

_____

_____

_____

_____

_____

# *Seizure Log*

| What Happened During the Seizure? | | | |
|---|:---:|---|:---:|
| The seizures started with the head | | The seizure started with the limbs | |
| The seizures started on the left / right | | My dog fell down | |
| Stiff body | | Floppy body | |
| Leg paddling | | Shaking | |
| Frothing / drooling | | Chewing movements | |
| Urination | | Defecation | |
| Weakness or twitching in one part of body | | Twitching on one side of face | |
| My dog could see | | My dog could hear | |
| Other: | | Other: | |

| What Happened After the Seizure? | | | |
|---|:---:|---|:---:|
| Wobbly | | Weakness in the limbs | |
| Blindness | | Sniffing | |
| Pacing | | Disorientated | |
| Sleepy / tired | | Clingy | |
| Behaviour change: Aggressive / Fearful | | Staring into space / standing in corners | |
| Other: | | Other: | |

| Possible Triggers | | | |
|---|:---:|---|:---:|
| Time of day | | Seizures were 'due' (regular interval) | |
| Missed / late medication | | Medication change | |
| Missed sleep | | Missed meal | |
| Exercise | | Temperature (too hot / cold) | |
| Sensory (Loud sounds / flashing lights etc.) | | Specific food. Please note: | |
| Other medication, treatments or supplements. Please note: | | Stressful event. Please describe: | |
| Other: | | Other: | |

# *Seizure Log*

Date: _____          Time: _____          Duration: _____

Location: _____

Seizure Type: _____

If this was a cluster how many seizures? _____

Was your dog: Asleep ☐   Awake ☐   Waking from sleep ☐

What happened during the seizure? _____

_____

_____

_____

What was happening around the time the seizure occurred?

_____

_____

_____

Was there an Aura or warning?  Yes ☐   No ☐   Describe: _____

_____

_____

Rescue medication if given: _____

Taken to vet? Yes ☐   No ☐   Detail: _____

How long did your dog take to recover? _____

Notes: _____

_____

_____

_____

_____

_____

# Seizure Log

| What Happened During the Seizure? | | | |
|---|---|---|---|
| The seizures started with the head | | The seizure started with the limbs | |
| The seizures started on the left / right | | My dog fell down | |
| Stiff body | | Floppy body | |
| Leg paddling | | Shaking | |
| Frothing / drooling | | Chewing movements | |
| Urination | | Defecation | |
| Weakness or twitching in one part of body | | Twitching on one side of face | |
| My dog could see | | My dog could hear | |
| Other: | | Other: | |

| What Happened After the Seizure? | | | |
|---|---|---|---|
| Wobbly | | Weakness in the limbs | |
| Blindness | | Sniffing | |
| Pacing | | Disorientated | |
| Sleepy / tired | | Clingy | |
| Behaviour change: Aggressive / Fearful | | Staring into space / standing in corners | |
| Other: | | Other: | |

| Possible Triggers | | | |
|---|---|---|---|
| Time of day | | Seizures were 'due' (regular interval) | |
| Missed / late medication | | Medication change | |
| Missed sleep | | Missed meal | |
| Exercise | | Temperature (too hot / cold) | |
| Sensory (Loud sounds / flashing lights etc.) | | Specific food. Please note: | |
| Other medication, treatments or supplements. Please note: | | Stressful event. Please describe: | |
| Other: | | Other: | |

# *Seizure Log*

Date: _____  Time: _____  Duration: _____

Location: _____

Seizure Type: _____

If this was a cluster how many seizures? _____

Was your dog: Asleep ☐  Awake ☐  Waking from sleep ☐

What happened during the seizure? _____

_____

_____

_____

What was happening around the time the seizure occurred?

_____

_____

_____

Was there an Aura or warning?  Yes ☐  No ☐  Describe: _____

_____

_____

Rescue medication if given: _____

Taken to vet? Yes ☐  No ☐  Detail: _____

How long did your dog take to recover? _____

Notes: _____

_____

_____

_____

_____

_____

# *Seizure Log*

| What Happened During the Seizure? | | | |
|---|---|---|---|
| The seizures started with the head | | The seizure started with the limbs | |
| The seizures started on the left / right | | My dog fell down | |
| Stiff body | | Floppy body | |
| Leg paddling | | Shaking | |
| Frothing / drooling | | Chewing movements | |
| Urination | | Defecation | |
| Weakness or twitching in one part of body | | Twitching on one side of face | |
| My dog could see | | My dog could hear | |
| Other: | | Other: | |

| What Happened After the Seizure? | | | |
|---|---|---|---|
| Wobbly | | Weakness in the limbs | |
| Blindness | | Sniffing | |
| Pacing | | Disorientated | |
| Sleepy / tired | | Clingy | |
| Behaviour change: Aggressive / Fearful | | Staring into space / standing in corners | |
| Other: | | Other: | |

| Possible Triggers | | | |
|---|---|---|---|
| Time of day | | Seizures were 'due' (regular interval) | |
| Missed / late medication | | Medication change | |
| Missed sleep | | Missed meal | |
| Exercise | | Temperature (too hot / cold) | |
| Sensory (Loud sounds / flashing lights etc.) | | Specific food. Please note: | |
| Other medication, treatments or supplements. Please note: | | Stressful event. Please describe: | |
| Other: | | Other: | |

# *Seizure Log*

Date: _____ Time: _____ Duration: _____

Location: _____

Seizure Type: _____

If this was a cluster how many seizures? _____

Was your dog: Asleep ☐   Awake ☐   Waking from sleep ☐

What happened during the seizure? _____

_____

_____

_____

What was happening around the time the seizure occurred?

_____

_____

_____

Was there an Aura or warning?  Yes ☐   No ☐   Describe: _____

_____

_____

Rescue medication if given: _____

Taken to vet? Yes ☐   No ☐   Detail: _____

How long did your dog take to recover? _____

Notes: _____

_____

_____

_____

_____

_____

# Seizure Log

| What Happened During the Seizure? | | | |
|---|---|---|---|
| The seizures started with the head | | The seizure started with the limbs | |
| The seizures started on the left / right | | My dog fell down | |
| Stiff body | | Floppy body | |
| Leg paddling | | Shaking | |
| Frothing / drooling | | Chewing movements | |
| Urination | | Defecation | |
| Weakness or twitching in one part of body | | Twitching on one side of face | |
| My dog could see | | My dog could hear | |
| Other: | | Other: | |

| What Happened After the Seizure? | | | |
|---|---|---|---|
| Wobbly | | Weakness in the limbs | |
| Blindness | | Sniffing | |
| Pacing | | Disorientated | |
| Sleepy / tired | | Clingy | |
| Behaviour change: Aggressive / Fearful | | Staring into space / standing in corners | |
| Other: | | Other: | |

| Possible Triggers | | | |
|---|---|---|---|
| Time of day | | Seizures were 'due' (regular interval) | |
| Missed / late medication | | Medication change | |
| Missed sleep | | Missed meal | |
| Exercise | | Temperature (too hot / cold) | |
| Sensory (Loud sounds / flashing lights etc.) | | Specific food. Please note: | |
| Other medication, treatments or supplements. Please note: | | Stressful event. Please describe: | |
| Other: | | Other: | |

# *Seizure Log*

Date: _____    Time: _____    Duration: _____

Location: _____

Seizure Type: _____

If this was a cluster how many seizures? _____

Was your dog: Asleep ☐   Awake ☐   Waking from sleep ☐

What happened during the seizure? _____

_____

_____

_____

What was happening around the time the seizure occurred?

_____

_____

_____

Was there an Aura or warning?   Yes ☐   No ☐   Describe: _____

_____

_____

Rescue medication if given: _____

Taken to vet? Yes ☐   No ☐   Detail: _____

How long did your dog take to recover? _____

_____

Notes: _____

_____

_____

_____

_____

_____

_____

# *Seizure Log*

| What Happened During the Seizure? | | | |
|---|---|---|---|
| The seizures started with the head | | The seizure started with the limbs | |
| The seizures started on the left / right | | My dog fell down | |
| Stiff body | | Floppy body | |
| Leg paddling | | Shaking | |
| Frothing / drooling | | Chewing movements | |
| Urination | | Defecation | |
| Weakness or twitching in one part of body | | Twitching on one side of face | |
| My dog could see | | My dog could hear | |
| Other: | | Other: | |

| What Happened After the Seizure? | | | |
|---|---|---|---|
| Wobbly | | Weakness in the limbs | |
| Blindness | | Sniffing | |
| Pacing | | Disorientated | |
| Sleepy / tired | | Clingy | |
| Behaviour change: Aggressive / Fearful | | Staring into space / standing in corners | |
| Other: | | Other: | |

| Possible Triggers | | | |
|---|---|---|---|
| Time of day | | Seizures were 'due' (regular interval) | |
| Missed / late medication | | Medication change | |
| Missed sleep | | Missed meal | |
| Exercise | | Temperature (too hot / cold) | |
| Sensory (Loud sounds / flashing lights etc.) | | Specific food. Please note: | |
| Other medication, treatments or supplements. Please note: | | Stressful event. Please describe: | |
| Other: | | Other: | |

# *Seizure Log*

Date: _____     Time: _____     Duration: _____

Location: _____

Seizure Type: _____

If this was a cluster how many seizures? _____

Was your dog: Asleep ☐   Awake ☐   Waking from sleep ☐

What happened during the seizure? _____

_____

_____

_____

What was happening around the time the seizure occurred?

_____

_____

_____

Was there an Aura or warning?  Yes ☐   No ☐   Describe: _____

_____

_____

Rescue medication if given: _____

Taken to vet? Yes ☐   No ☐   Detail: _____

How long did your dog take to recover? _____

Notes: _____

_____

_____

_____

_____

_____

# *Seizure Log*

## What Happened During the Seizure?

| | | |
|---|---|---|
| The seizures started with the head | The seizure started with the limbs | |
| The seizures started on the left / right | My dog fell down | |
| Stiff body | Floppy body | |
| Leg paddling | Shaking | |
| Frothing / drooling | Chewing movements | |
| Urination | Defecation | |
| Weakness or twitching in one part of body | Twitching on one side of face | |
| My dog could see | My dog could hear | |
| Other: | Other: | |

## What Happened After the Seizure?

| | | |
|---|---|---|
| Wobbly | Weakness in the limbs | |
| Blindness | Sniffing | |
| Pacing | Disorientated | |
| Sleepy / tired | Clingy | |
| Behaviour change: Aggressive / Fearful | Staring into space / standing in corners | |
| Other: | Other: | |

## Possible Triggers

| | | |
|---|---|---|
| Time of day | Seizures were 'due' (regular interval) | |
| Missed / late medication | Medication change | |
| Missed sleep | Missed meal | |
| Exercise | Temperature (too hot / cold) | |
| Sensory (Loud sounds / flashing lights etc.) | Specific food. Please note: | |
| Other medication, treatments or supplements. Please note: | Stressful event. Please describe: | |
| Other: | Other: | |

# *Seizure Log*

Date: _____  Time: _____  Duration: _____

Location: _____

Seizure Type: _____

If this was a cluster how many seizures? _____

Was your dog: Asleep ☐  Awake ☐  Waking from sleep ☐

What happened during the seizure? _____

_____

_____

_____

What was happening around the time the seizure occurred?

_____

_____

_____

Was there an Aura or warning?  Yes ☐  No ☐  Describe: _____

_____

_____

Rescue medication if given: _____

Taken to vet? Yes ☐  No ☐  Detail: _____

How long did your dog take to recover? _____

Notes: _____

_____

_____

_____

_____

_____

# *Seizure Log*

| What Happened During the Seizure? | | | |
|---|---|---|---|
| The seizures started with the head | | The seizure started with the limbs | |
| The seizures started on the left / right | | My dog fell down | |
| Stiff body | | Floppy body | |
| Leg paddling | | Shaking | |
| Frothing / drooling | | Chewing movements | |
| Urination | | Defecation | |
| Weakness or twitching in one part of body | | Twitching on one side of face | |
| My dog could see | | My dog could hear | |
| Other: | | Other: | |

| What Happened After the Seizure? | | | |
|---|---|---|---|
| Wobbly | | Weakness in the limbs | |
| Blindness | | Sniffing | |
| Pacing | | Disorientated | |
| Sleepy / tired | | Clingy | |
| Behaviour change: Aggressive / Fearful | | Staring into space / standing in corners | |
| Other: | | Other: | |

| Possible Triggers | | | |
|---|---|---|---|
| Time of day | | Seizures were 'due' (regular interval) | |
| Missed / late medication | | Medication change | |
| Missed sleep | | Missed meal | |
| Exercise | | Temperature (too hot / cold) | |
| Sensory (Loud sounds / flashing lights etc.) | | Specific food. Please note: | |
| Other medication, treatments or supplements. Please note: | | Stressful event. Please describe: | |
| Other: | | Other: | |

# *Seizure Log*

Date: _____  Time: _____  Duration: _____

Location: _____

Seizure Type: _____

If this was a cluster how many seizures? _____

Was your dog: Asleep ☐  Awake ☐  Waking from sleep ☐

What happened during the seizure? _____

_____

_____

What was happening around the time the seizure occurred?

_____

_____

Was there an Aura or warning?  Yes ☐  No ☐  Describe: _____

_____

Rescue medication if given: _____

Taken to vet? Yes ☐  No ☐  Detail: _____

How long did your dog take to recover? _____

Notes:

_____

_____

_____

_____

_____

# *Seizure Log*

| What Happened During the Seizure? | | | |
|---|---|---|---|
| The seizures started with the head | | The seizure started with the limbs | |
| The seizures started on the left / right | | My dog fell down | |
| Stiff body | | Floppy body | |
| Leg paddling | | Shaking | |
| Frothing / drooling | | Chewing movements | |
| Urination | | Defecation | |
| Weakness or twitching in one part of body | | Twitching on one side of face | |
| My dog could see | | My dog could hear | |
| Other: | | Other: | |

| What Happened After the Seizure? | | | |
|---|---|---|---|
| Wobbly | | Weakness in the limbs | |
| Blindness | | Sniffing | |
| Pacing | | Disorientated | |
| Sleepy / tired | | Clingy | |
| Behaviour change: Aggressive / Fearful | | Staring into space / standing in corners | |
| Other: | | Other: | |

| Possible Triggers | | | |
|---|---|---|---|
| Time of day | | Seizures were 'due' (regular interval) | |
| Missed / late medication | | Medication change | |
| Missed sleep | | Missed meal | |
| Exercise | | Temperature (too hot / cold) | |
| Sensory (Loud sounds / flashing lights etc.) | | Specific food. Please note: | |
| Other medication, treatments or supplements. Please note: | | Stressful event. Please describe: | |
| Other: | | Other: | |

# *Seizure Log*

Date: _____  Time: _____  Duration: _____

Location: _____

Seizure Type: _____

If this was a cluster how many seizures? _____

Was your dog: Asleep ☐  Awake ☐  Waking from sleep ☐

What happened during the seizure? _____

_____

_____

_____

What was happening around the time the seizure occurred?

_____

_____

Was there an Aura or warning?  Yes ☐  No ☐  Describe: _____

_____

_____

Rescue medication if given: _____

Taken to vet? Yes ☐  No ☐  Detail: _____

How long did your dog take to recover? _____

Notes: _____

_____

_____

_____

_____

_____

# *Seizure Log*

| What Happened During the Seizure? | | |
|---|---|---|
| The seizures started with the head | The seizure started with the limbs | |
| The seizures started on the left / right | My dog fell down | |
| Stiff body | Floppy body | |
| Leg paddling | Shaking | |
| Frothing / drooling | Chewing movements | |
| Urination | Defecation | |
| Weakness or twitching in one part of body | Twitching on one side of face | |
| My dog could see | My dog could hear | |
| Other: | Other: | |

| What Happened After the Seizure? | | |
|---|---|---|
| Wobbly | Weakness in the limbs | |
| Blindness | Sniffing | |
| Pacing | Disorientated | |
| Sleepy / tired | Clingy | |
| Behaviour change: Aggressive / Fearful | Staring into space / standing in corners | |
| Other: | Other: | |

| Possible Triggers | | |
|---|---|---|
| Time of day | Seizures were 'due' (regular interval) | |
| Missed / late medication | Medication change | |
| Missed sleep | Missed meal | |
| Exercise | Temperature (too hot / cold) | |
| Sensory (Loud sounds / flashing lights etc.) | Specific food. Please note: | |
| Other medication, treatments or supplements. Please note: | Stressful event. Please describe: | |
| Other: | Other: | |

# *Seizure Log*

Date: _____ Time: _____ Duration: _____

Location: _____

Seizure Type: _____

If this was a cluster how many seizures? _____

Was your dog: Asleep ☐ Awake ☐ Waking from sleep ☐

What happened during the seizure? _____

_____

_____

_____

What was happening around the time the seizure occurred?

_____

_____

_____

Was there an Aura or warning? Yes ☐ No ☐ Describe: _____

_____

_____

Rescue medication if given: _____

Taken to vet? Yes ☐ No ☐ Detail: _____

How long did your dog take to recover? _____

_____

Notes: _____

_____

_____

_____

_____

_____

_____

# *Seizure Log*

## What Happened During the Seizure?

| | | |
|---|---|---|
| The seizures started with the head | The seizure started with the limbs | |
| The seizures started on the left / right | My dog fell down | |
| Stiff body | Floppy body | |
| Leg paddling | Shaking | |
| Frothing / drooling | Chewing movements | |
| Urination | Defecation | |
| Weakness or twitching in one part of body | Twitching on one side of face | |
| My dog could see | My dog could hear | |
| Other: | Other: | |

## What Happened After the Seizure?

| | | |
|---|---|---|
| Wobbly | Weakness in the limbs | |
| Blindness | Sniffing | |
| Pacing | Disorientated | |
| Sleepy / tired | Clingy | |
| Behaviour change: Aggressive / Fearful | Staring into space / standing in corners | |
| Other: | Other: | |

## Possible Triggers

| | | |
|---|---|---|
| Time of day | Seizures were 'due' (regular interval) | |
| Missed / late medication | Medication change | |
| Missed sleep | Missed meal | |
| Exercise | Temperature (too hot / cold) | |
| Sensory (Loud sounds / flashing lights etc.) | Specific food. Please note: | |
| Other medication, treatments or supplements. Please note: | Stressful event. Please describe: | |
| Other: | Other: | |

## *Seizure Log*

Date: _____     Time: _____     Duration: _____

Location: .................................................................................................................................

Seizure Type: .........................................................................................................................

If this was a cluster how many seizures? ........................................................................

Was your dog: Asleep ☐   Awake ☐   Waking from sleep ☐

What happened during the seizure? .................................................................................

.............................................................................................................................................

.............................................................................................................................................

.............................................................................................................................................

What was happening around the time the seizure occurred?

.............................................................................................................................................

.............................................................................................................................................

.............................................................................................................................................

Was there an Aura or warning?  Yes ☐   No ☐   Describe: ............................................

.............................................................................................................................................

.............................................................................................................................................

Rescue medication if given: _____

Taken to vet? Yes ☐   No ☐   Detail: ............................................................................

How long did your dog take to recover? .........................................................................

Notes: ...................................................................................................................................

.............................................................................................................................................

.............................................................................................................................................

.............................................................................................................................................

.............................................................................................................................................

.............................................................................................................................................

# *Seizure Log*

| What Happened During the Seizure? | | | |
|---|---|---|---|
| The seizures started with the head | | The seizure started with the limbs | |
| The seizures started on the left / right | | My dog fell down | |
| Stiff body | | Floppy body | |
| Leg paddling | | Shaking | |
| Frothing / drooling | | Chewing movements | |
| Urination | | Defecation | |
| Weakness or twitching in one part of body | | Twitching on one side of face | |
| My dog could see | | My dog could hear | |
| Other: | | Other: | |

| What Happened After the Seizure? | | | |
|---|---|---|---|
| Wobbly | | Weakness in the limbs | |
| Blindness | | Sniffing | |
| Pacing | | Disorientated | |
| Sleepy / tired | | Clingy | |
| Behaviour change: Aggressive / Fearful | | Staring into space / standing in corners | |
| Other: | | Other: | |

| Possible Triggers | | | |
|---|---|---|---|
| Time of day | | Seizures were 'due' (regular interval) | |
| Missed / late medication | | Medication change | |
| Missed sleep | | Missed meal | |
| Exercise | | Temperature (too hot / cold) | |
| Sensory (Loud sounds / flashing lights etc.) | | Specific food. Please note: | |
| Other medication, treatments or supplements. Please note: | | Stressful event. Please describe: | |
| Other: | | Other: | |

# *Seizure Log*

Date: _____ Time: _____ Duration: _____

Location: _____

Seizure Type: _____

If this was a cluster how many seizures? _____

Was your dog: Asleep ☐  Awake ☐  Waking from sleep ☐

What happened during the seizure? _____

_____

_____

What was happening around the time the seizure occurred?

_____

_____

Was there an Aura or warning?  Yes ☐  No ☐  Describe: _____

_____

Rescue medication if given: _____

Taken to vet? Yes ☐  No ☐  Detail: _____

How long did your dog take to recover? _____

Notes:

_____

_____

_____

_____

_____

# Seizure Log

| What Happened During the Seizure? | | | |
|---|---|---|---|
| The seizures started with the head | | The seizure started with the limbs | |
| The seizures started on the left / right | | My dog fell down | |
| Stiff body | | Floppy body | |
| Leg paddling | | Shaking | |
| Frothing / drooling | | Chewing movements | |
| Urination | | Defecation | |
| Weakness or twitching in one part of body | | Twitching on one side of face | |
| My dog could see | | My dog could hear | |
| Other: | | Other: | |

| What Happened After the Seizure? | | | |
|---|---|---|---|
| Wobbly | | Weakness in the limbs | |
| Blindness | | Sniffing | |
| Pacing | | Disorientated | |
| Sleepy / tired | | Clingy | |
| Behaviour change: Aggressive / Fearful | | Staring into space / standing in corners | |
| Other: | | Other: | |

| Possible Triggers | | | |
|---|---|---|---|
| Time of day | | Seizures were 'due' (regular interval) | |
| Missed / late medication | | Medication change | |
| Missed sleep | | Missed meal | |
| Exercise | | Temperature (too hot / cold) | |
| Sensory (Loud sounds / flashing lights etc.) | | Specific food. Please note: | |
| Other medication, treatments or supplements. Please note: | | Stressful event. Please describe: | |
| Other: | | Other: | |

# *Seizure Log*

Date: _____ Time: _____ Duration: _____

Location: _____

Seizure Type: _____

If this was a cluster how many seizures? _____

Was your dog: Asleep ☐  Awake ☐  Waking from sleep ☐

What happened during the seizure? _____

_____

_____

_____

What was happening around the time the seizure occurred?

_____

_____

_____

Was there an Aura or warning?  Yes ☐  No ☐  Describe: _____

_____

_____

Rescue medication if given: _____

Taken to vet? Yes ☐  No ☐  Detail: _____

How long did your dog take to recover? _____

Notes: _____

_____

_____

_____

_____

_____

_____

# Seizure Log

| What Happened During the Seizure? | | | |
|---|---|---|---|
| The seizures started with the head | | The seizure started with the limbs | |
| The seizures started on the left / right | | My dog fell down | |
| Stiff body | | Floppy body | |
| Leg paddling | | Shaking | |
| Frothing / drooling | | Chewing movements | |
| Urination | | Defecation | |
| Weakness or twitching in one part of body | | Twitching on one side of face | |
| My dog could see | | My dog could hear | |
| Other: | | Other: | |

| What Happened After the Seizure? | | | |
|---|---|---|---|
| Wobbly | | Weakness in the limbs | |
| Blindness | | Sniffing | |
| Pacing | | Disorientated | |
| Sleepy / tired | | Clingy | |
| Behaviour change: Aggressive / Fearful | | Staring into space / standing in corners | |
| Other: | | Other: | |

| Possible Triggers | | | |
|---|---|---|---|
| Time of day | | Seizures were 'due' (regular interval) | |
| Missed / late medication | | Medication change | |
| Missed sleep | | Missed meal | |
| Exercise | | Temperature (too hot / cold) | |
| Sensory (Loud sounds / flashing lights etc.) | | Specific food. Please note: | |
| Other medication, treatments or supplements. Please note: | | Stressful event. Please describe: | |
| Other: | | Other: | |

# *Seizure Log*

Date: _____ Time: _____ Duration: _____

Location: _____

Seizure Type: _____

If this was a cluster how many seizures? _____

Was your dog: Asleep ☐   Awake ☐   Waking from sleep ☐

What happened during the seizure?
_____
_____
_____

What was happening around the time the seizure occurred?
_____
_____
_____

Was there an Aura or warning?  Yes ☐   No ☐   Describe: _____
_____

Rescue medication if given: _____

Taken to vet? Yes ☐   No ☐   Detail: _____

How long did your dog take to recover? _____

Notes:
_____
_____
_____
_____
_____
_____

# *Seizure Log*

| What Happened During the Seizure? | | | |
|---|---|---|---|
| The seizures started with the head | | The seizure started with the limbs | |
| The seizures started on the left / right | | My dog fell down | |
| Stiff body | | Floppy body | |
| Leg paddling | | Shaking | |
| Frothing / drooling | | Chewing movements | |
| Urination | | Defecation | |
| Weakness or twitching in one part of body | | Twitching on one side of face | |
| My dog could see | | My dog could hear | |
| Other: | | Other: | |

| What Happened After the Seizure? | | | |
|---|---|---|---|
| Wobbly | | Weakness in the limbs | |
| Blindness | | Sniffing | |
| Pacing | | Disorientated | |
| Sleepy / tired | | Clingy | |
| Behaviour change: Aggressive / Fearful | | Staring into space / standing in corners | |
| Other: | | Other: | |

| Possible Triggers | | | |
|---|---|---|---|
| Time of day | | Seizures were 'due' (regular interval) | |
| Missed / late medication | | Medication change | |
| Missed sleep | | Missed meal | |
| Exercise | | Temperature (too hot / cold) | |
| Sensory (Loud sounds / flashing lights etc.) | | Specific food. Please note: | |
| Other medication, treatments or supplements. Please note: | | Stressful event. Please describe: | |
| Other: | | Other: | |

# *Seizure Log*

Date: _____ Time: _____ Duration: _____

Location: _____

Seizure Type: _____

If this was a cluster how many seizures? _____

Was your dog: Asleep ☐ Awake ☐ Waking from sleep ☐

What happened during the seizure?
_____
_____
_____
_____

What was happening around the time the seizure occurred?
_____
_____
_____

Was there an Aura or warning? Yes ☐ No ☐ Describe: _____
_____
_____

Rescue medication if given: _____

Taken to vet? Yes ☐ No ☐ Detail: _____

How long did your dog take to recover? _____

Notes:
_____
_____
_____
_____
_____
_____

# *Seizure Log*

| What Happened During the Seizure? | | | |
|---|---|---|---|
| The seizures started with the head | | The seizure started with the limbs | |
| The seizures started on the left / right | | My dog fell down | |
| Stiff body | | Floppy body | |
| Leg paddling | | Shaking | |
| Frothing / drooling | | Chewing movements | |
| Urination | | Defecation | |
| Weakness or twitching in one part of body | | Twitching on one side of face | |
| My dog could see | | My dog could hear | |
| Other: | | Other: | |

| What Happened After the Seizure? | | | |
|---|---|---|---|
| Wobbly | | Weakness in the limbs | |
| Blindness | | Sniffing | |
| Pacing | | Disorientated | |
| Sleepy / tired | | Clingy | |
| Behaviour change: Aggressive / Fearful | | Staring into space / standing in corners | |
| Other: | | Other: | |

| Possible Triggers | | | |
|---|---|---|---|
| Time of day | | Seizures were 'due' (regular interval) | |
| Missed / late medication | | Medication change | |
| Missed sleep | | Missed meal | |
| Exercise | | Temperature (too hot / cold) | |
| Sensory (Loud sounds / flashing lights etc.) | | Specific food. Please note: | |
| Other medication, treatments or supplements. Please note: | | Stressful event. Please describe: | |
| Other: | | Other: | |

# *Seizure Log*

Date: _____  Time: _____  Duration: _____

Location: _____

Seizure Type: _____

If this was a cluster how many seizures? _____

Was your dog: Asleep ☐  Awake ☐  Waking from sleep ☐

What happened during the seizure?

_____

_____

_____

What was happening around the time the seizure occurred?

_____

_____

Was there an Aura or warning?  Yes ☐  No ☐  Describe: _____

_____

Rescue medication if given: _____

Taken to vet? Yes ☐  No ☐  Detail: _____

How long did your dog take to recover? _____

Notes:

_____

_____

_____

_____

_____

# *Seizure Log*

| What Happened During the Seizure? | | | |
|---|---|---|---|
| The seizures started with the head | | The seizure started with the limbs | |
| The seizures started on the left / right | | My dog fell down | |
| Stiff body | | Floppy body | |
| Leg paddling | | Shaking | |
| Frothing / drooling | | Chewing movements | |
| Urination | | Defecation | |
| Weakness or twitching in one part of body | | Twitching on one side of face | |
| My dog could see | | My dog could hear | |
| Other: | | Other: | |

| What Happened After the Seizure? | | | |
|---|---|---|---|
| Wobbly | | Weakness in the limbs | |
| Blindness | | Sniffing | |
| Pacing | | Disorientated | |
| Sleepy / tired | | Clingy | |
| Behaviour change: Aggressive / Fearful | | Staring into space / standing in corners | |
| Other: | | Other: | |

| Possible Triggers | | | |
|---|---|---|---|
| Time of day | | Seizures were 'due' (regular interval) | |
| Missed / late medication | | Medication change | |
| Missed sleep | | Missed meal | |
| Exercise | | Temperature (too hot / cold) | |
| Sensory (Loud sounds / flashing lights etc.) | | Specific food. Please note: | |
| Other medication, treatments or supplements. Please note: | | Stressful event. Please describe: | |
| Other: | | Other: | |

# *Seizure Log*

Date: _____ Time: _____ Duration: _____

Location: _____

Seizure Type: _____

If this was a cluster how many seizures? _____

Was your dog: Asleep ☐  Awake ☐  Waking from sleep ☐

What happened during the seizure? _____

_____

_____

What was happening around the time the seizure occurred?

_____

_____

Was there an Aura or warning?  Yes ☐  No ☐  Describe: _____

_____

Rescue medication if given: _____

Taken to vet? Yes ☐  No ☐  Detail: _____

How long did your dog take to recover? _____

Notes: _____

_____

_____

_____

_____

# *Seizure Log*

| What Happened During the Seizure? | | | |
|---|---|---|---|
| The seizures started with the head | | The seizure started with the limbs | |
| The seizures started on the left / right | | My dog fell down | |
| Stiff body | | Floppy body | |
| Leg paddling | | Shaking | |
| Frothing / drooling | | Chewing movements | |
| Urination | | Defecation | |
| Weakness or twitching in one part of body | | Twitching on one side of face | |
| My dog could see | | My dog could hear | |
| Other: | | Other: | |

| What Happened After the Seizure? | | | |
|---|---|---|---|
| Wobbly | | Weakness in the limbs | |
| Blindness | | Sniffing | |
| Pacing | | Disorientated | |
| Sleepy / tired | | Clingy | |
| Behaviour change: Aggressive / Fearful | | Staring into space / standing in corners | |
| Other: | | Other: | |

| Possible Triggers | | | |
|---|---|---|---|
| Time of day | | Seizures were 'due' (regular interval) | |
| Missed / late medication | | Medication change | |
| Missed sleep | | Missed meal | |
| Exercise | | Temperature (too hot / cold) | |
| Sensory (Loud sounds / flashing lights etc.) | | Specific food. Please note: | |
| Other medication, treatments or supplements. Please note: | | Stressful event. Please describe: | |
| Other: | | Other: | |

61

# *Seizure Log*

Date: _____    Time: _____    Duration: _____

Location: _____

Seizure Type: _____

If this was a cluster how many seizures? _____

Was your dog: Asleep ☐   Awake ☐   Waking from sleep ☐

What happened during the seizure? _____

_____

_____

_____

What was happening around the time the seizure occurred? _____

_____

_____

_____

Was there an Aura or warning?  Yes ☐   No ☐   Describe: _____

_____

_____

Rescue medication if given: _____

Taken to vet? Yes ☐   No ☐   Detail: _____

How long did your dog take to recover? _____

Notes: _____

_____

_____

_____

_____

# *Seizure Log*

| What Happened During the Seizure? | | | |
|---|---|---|---|
| The seizures started with the head | | The seizure started with the limbs | |
| The seizures started on the left / right | | My dog fell down | |
| Stiff body | | Floppy body | |
| Leg paddling | | Shaking | |
| Frothing / drooling | | Chewing movements | |
| Urination | | Defecation | |
| Weakness or twitching in one part of body | | Twitching on one side of face | |
| My dog could see | | My dog could hear | |
| Other: | | Other: | |

| What Happened After the Seizure? | | | |
|---|---|---|---|
| Wobbly | | Weakness in the limbs | |
| Blindness | | Sniffing | |
| Pacing | | Disorientated | |
| Sleepy / tired | | Clingy | |
| Behaviour change: Aggressive / Fearful | | Staring into space / standing in corners | |
| Other: | | Other: | |

| Possible Triggers | | | |
|---|---|---|---|
| Time of day | | Seizures were 'due' (regular interval) | |
| Missed / late medication | | Medication change | |
| Missed sleep | | Missed meal | |
| Exercise | | Temperature (too hot / cold) | |
| Sensory (Loud sounds / flashing lights etc.) | | Specific food. Please note: | |
| Other medication, treatments or supplements. Please note: | | Stressful event. Please describe: | |
| Other: | | Other: | |

# *Seizure Log*

Date: _____    Time: _____    Duration: _____

Location: _____

Seizure Type: _____

If this was a cluster how many seizures? _____

Was your dog: Asleep ☐  Awake ☐  Waking from sleep ☐

What happened during the seizure?

_____

_____

_____

What was happening around the time the seizure occurred?

_____

_____

_____

Was there an Aura or warning?  Yes ☐  No ☐  Describe: _____

_____

_____

Rescue medication if given: _____

Taken to vet? Yes ☐  No ☐  Detail: _____

How long did your dog take to recover? _____

Notes:

_____

_____

_____

_____

_____

_____

# *Seizure Log*

| What Happened During the Seizure? | | | |
|---|---|---|---|
| The seizures started with the head | | The seizure started with the limbs | |
| The seizures started on the left / right | | My dog fell down | |
| Stiff body | | Floppy body | |
| Leg paddling | | Shaking | |
| Frothing / drooling | | Chewing movements | |
| Urination | | Defecation | |
| Weakness or twitching in one part of body | | Twitching on one side of face | |
| My dog could see | | My dog could hear | |
| Other: | | Other: | |

| What Happened After the Seizure? | | | |
|---|---|---|---|
| Wobbly | | Weakness in the limbs | |
| Blindness | | Sniffing | |
| Pacing | | Disorientated | |
| Sleepy / tired | | Clingy | |
| Behaviour change: Aggressive / Fearful | | Staring into space / standing in corners | |
| Other: | | Other: | |

| Possible Triggers | | | |
|---|---|---|---|
| Time of day | | Seizures were 'due' (regular interval) | |
| Missed / late medication | | Medication change | |
| Missed sleep | | Missed meal | |
| Exercise | | Temperature (too hot / cold) | |
| Sensory (Loud sounds / flashing lights etc.) | | Specific food. Please note: | |
| Other medication, treatments or supplements. Please note: | | Stressful event. Please describe: | |
| Other: | | Other: | |

# *Seizure Log*

Date: _____  Time: _____  Duration: _____

Location: _____

Seizure Type: _____

If this was a cluster how many seizures? _____

Was your dog: Asleep ☐  Awake ☐  Waking from sleep ☐

What happened during the seizure? _____

_____

_____

_____

What was happening around the time the seizure occurred?

_____

_____

_____

Was there an Aura or warning?  Yes ☐  No ☐  Describe: _____

_____

_____

Rescue medication if given: _____

Taken to vet? Yes ☐  No ☐  Detail: _____

How long did your dog take to recover? _____

Notes: _____

_____

_____

_____

_____

_____

_____

# *Seizure Log*

| What Happened During the Seizure? | | | |
|---|---|---|---|
| The seizures started with the head | | The seizure started with the limbs | |
| The seizures started on the left / right | | My dog fell down | |
| Stiff body | | Floppy body | |
| Leg paddling | | Shaking | |
| Frothing / drooling | | Chewing movements | |
| Urination | | Defecation | |
| Weakness or twitching in one part of body | | Twitching on one side of face | |
| My dog could see | | My dog could hear | |
| Other: | | Other: | |

| What Happened After the Seizure? | | | |
|---|---|---|---|
| Wobbly | | Weakness in the limbs | |
| Blindness | | Sniffing | |
| Pacing | | Disorientated | |
| Sleepy / tired | | Clingy | |
| Behaviour change: Aggressive / Fearful | | Staring into space / standing in corners | |
| Other: | | Other: | |

| Possible Triggers | | | |
|---|---|---|---|
| Time of day | | Seizures were 'due' (regular interval) | |
| Missed / late medication | | Medication change | |
| Missed sleep | | Missed meal | |
| Exercise | | Temperature (too hot / cold) | |
| Sensory (Loud sounds / flashing lights etc.) | | Specific food. Please note: | |
| Other medication, treatments or supplements. Please note: | | Stressful event. Please describe: | |
| Other: | | Other: | |

67

# *Seizure Log*

Date: _____ Time: _____ Duration: _____

Location: _____

Seizure Type: _____

If this was a cluster how many seizures? _____

Was your dog: Asleep ☐  Awake ☐  Waking from sleep ☐

What happened during the seizure? _____

_____

_____

What was happening around the time the seizure occurred?

_____

_____

Was there an Aura or warning?  Yes ☐  No ☐  Describe: _____

_____

Rescue medication if given: _____

Taken to vet? Yes ☐  No ☐  Detail: _____

How long did your dog take to recover? _____

Notes: _____

_____

_____

_____

_____

_____

# *Seizure Log*

## What Happened During the Seizure?

| | | | |
|---|---|---|---|
| The seizures started with the head | | The seizure started with the limbs | |
| The seizures started on the left / right | | My dog fell down | |
| Stiff body | | Floppy body | |
| Leg paddling | | Shaking | |
| Frothing / drooling | | Chewing movements | |
| Urination | | Defecation | |
| Weakness or twitching in one part of body | | Twitching on one side of face | |
| My dog could see | | My dog could hear | |
| Other: | | Other: | |

## What Happened After the Seizure?

| | | | |
|---|---|---|---|
| Wobbly | | Weakness in the limbs | |
| Blindness | | Sniffing | |
| Pacing | | Disorientated | |
| Sleepy / tired | | Clingy | |
| Behaviour change: Aggressive / Fearful | | Staring into space / standing in corners | |
| Other: | | Other: | |

## Possible Triggers

| | | | |
|---|---|---|---|
| Time of day | | Seizures were 'due' (regular interval) | |
| Missed / late medication | | Medication change | |
| Missed sleep | | Missed meal | |
| Exercise | | Temperature (too hot / cold) | |
| Sensory (Loud sounds / flashing lights etc.) | | Specific food. Please note: | |
| Other medication, treatments or supplements. Please note: | | Stressful event. Please describe: | |
| Other: | | Other: | |

# *Seizure Log*

Date: _____   Time: _____   Duration: _____

Location: .................................................................................................

Seizure Type: ...........................................................................................

If this was a cluster how many seizures? ...............................................

Was your dog: Asleep ☐  Awake ☐  Waking from sleep ☐

What happened during the seizure? ........................................................

.................................................................................................................

.................................................................................................................

.................................................................................................................

What was happening around the time the seizure occurred?

.................................................................................................................

.................................................................................................................

.................................................................................................................

Was there an Aura or warning?  Yes ☐  No ☐  Describe: ...................

.................................................................................................................

.................................................................................................................

Rescue medication if given: ....................................................................

Taken to vet? Yes ☐  No ☐  Detail: _____

How long did your dog take to recover? .................................................

Notes: ......................................................................................................

.................................................................................................................

.................................................................................................................

.................................................................................................................

.................................................................................................................

.................................................................................................................

# *Seizure Log*

| What Happened During the Seizure? | | | |
|---|---|---|---|
| The seizures started with the head | | The seizure started with the limbs | |
| The seizures started on the left / right | | My dog fell down | |
| Stiff body | | Floppy body | |
| Leg paddling | | Shaking | |
| Frothing / drooling | | Chewing movements | |
| Urination | | Defecation | |
| Weakness or twitching in one part of body | | Twitching on one side of face | |
| My dog could see | | My dog could hear | |
| Other: | | Other: | |

| What Happened After the Seizure? | | | |
|---|---|---|---|
| Wobbly | | Weakness in the limbs | |
| Blindness | | Sniffing | |
| Pacing | | Disorientated | |
| Sleepy / tired | | Clingy | |
| Behaviour change: Aggressive / Fearful | | Staring into space / standing in corners | |
| Other: | | Other: | |

| Possible Triggers | | | |
|---|---|---|---|
| Time of day | | Seizures were 'due' (regular interval) | |
| Missed / late medication | | Medication change | |
| Missed sleep | | Missed meal | |
| Exercise | | Temperature (too hot / cold) | |
| Sensory (Loud sounds / flashing lights etc.) | | Specific food. Please note: | |
| Other medication, treatments or supplements. Please note: | | Stressful event. Please describe: | |
| Other: | | Other: | |

# *Seizure Log*

Date: _____ Time: _____ Duration: _____

Location: _____

Seizure Type: _____

If this was a cluster how many seizures? _____

Was your dog: Asleep ☐  Awake ☐  Waking from sleep ☐

What happened during the seizure? _____

_____

_____

What was happening around the time the seizure occurred? _____

_____

_____

Was there an Aura or warning?  Yes ☐  No ☐  Describe: _____

_____

Rescue medication if given: _____

Taken to vet? Yes ☐  No ☐  Detail: _____

How long did your dog take to recover? _____

Notes: _____

_____

_____

_____

_____

_____

# *Seizure Log*

| What Happened During the Seizure? | | | | |
|---|---|---|---|---|
| The seizures started with the head | | The seizure started with the limbs | | |
| The seizures started on the left / right | | My dog fell down | | |
| Stiff body | | Floppy body | | |
| Leg paddling | | Shaking | | |
| Frothing / drooling | | Chewing movements | | |
| Urination | | Defecation | | |
| Weakness or twitching in one part of body | | Twitching on one side of face | | |
| My dog could see | | My dog could hear | | |
| Other: | | Other: | | |

| What Happened After the Seizure? | | | | |
|---|---|---|---|---|
| Wobbly | | Weakness in the limbs | | |
| Blindness | | Sniffing | | |
| Pacing | | Disorientated | | |
| Sleepy / tired | | Clingy | | |
| Behaviour change: Aggressive / Fearful | | Staring into space / standing in corners | | |
| Other: | | Other: | | |

| Possible Triggers | | | | |
|---|---|---|---|---|
| Time of day | | Seizures were 'due' (regular interval) | | |
| Missed / late medication | | Medication change | | |
| Missed sleep | | Missed meal | | |
| Exercise | | Temperature (too hot / cold) | | |
| Sensory (Loud sounds / flashing lights etc.) | | Specific food. Please note: | | |
| Other medication, treatments or supplements. Please note: | | Stressful event. Please describe: | | |
| Other: | | Other: | | |

## *Seizure Log*

Date: _____ Time: _____ Duration: _____

Location: _____

Seizure Type: _____

If this was a cluster how many seizures? _____

Was your dog: Asleep ☐ Awake ☐ Waking from sleep ☐

What happened during the seizure?

_____

_____

_____

What was happening around the time the seizure occurred?

_____

_____

Was there an Aura or warning? Yes ☐ No ☐ Describe: _____

_____

Rescue medication if given: _____

Taken to vet? Yes ☐ No ☐ Detail: _____

How long did your dog take to recover? _____

Notes:

_____

_____

_____

_____

_____

# *Seizure Log*

| What Happened During the Seizure? | | | |
|---|---|---|---|
| The seizures started with the head | | The seizure started with the limbs | |
| The seizures started on the left / right | | My dog fell down | |
| Stiff body | | Floppy body | |
| Leg paddling | | Shaking | |
| Frothing / drooling | | Chewing movements | |
| Urination | | Defecation | |
| Weakness or twitching in one part of body | | Twitching on one side of face | |
| My dog could see | | My dog could hear | |
| Other: | | Other: | |

| What Happened After the Seizure? | | | |
|---|---|---|---|
| Wobbly | | Weakness in the limbs | |
| Blindness | | Sniffing | |
| Pacing | | Disorientated | |
| Sleepy / tired | | Clingy | |
| Behaviour change: Aggressive / Fearful | | Staring into space / standing in corners | |
| Other: | | Other: | |

| Possible Triggers | | | |
|---|---|---|---|
| Time of day | | Seizures were 'due' (regular interval) | |
| Missed / late medication | | Medication change | |
| Missed sleep | | Missed meal | |
| Exercise | | Temperature (too hot / cold) | |
| Sensory (Loud sounds / flashing lights etc.) | | Specific food. Please note: | |
| Other medication, treatments or supplements. Please note: | | Stressful event. Please describe: | |
| Other: | | Other: | |

75

## *Seizure Log*

Date: _____  Time: _____  Duration: _____

Location: _____

Seizure Type: _____

If this was a cluster how many seizures? _____

Was your dog: Asleep ☐  Awake ☐  Waking from sleep ☐

What happened during the seizure?

_____

_____

What was happening around the time the seizure occurred?

_____

_____

Was there an Aura or warning?  Yes ☐  No ☐  Describe: _____

_____

_____

Rescue medication if given: _____

Taken to vet? Yes ☐  No ☐  Detail: _____

How long did your dog take to recover? _____

Notes:

_____

_____

_____

_____

_____

_____

# *Seizure Log*

## What Happened During the Seizure?

| | | | |
|---|---|---|---|
| The seizures started with the head | | The seizure started with the limbs | |
| The seizures started on the left / right | | My dog fell down | |
| Stiff body | | Floppy body | |
| Leg paddling | | Shaking | |
| Frothing / drooling | | Chewing movements | |
| Urination | | Defecation | |
| Weakness or twitching in one part of body | | Twitching on one side of face | |
| My dog could see | | My dog could hear | |
| Other: | | Other: | |

## What Happened After the Seizure?

| | | | |
|---|---|---|---|
| Wobbly | | Weakness in the limbs | |
| Blindness | | Sniffing | |
| Pacing | | Disorientated | |
| Sleepy / tired | | Clingy | |
| Behaviour change: Aggressive / Fearful | | Staring into space / standing in corners | |
| Other: | | Other: | |

## Possible Triggers

| | | | |
|---|---|---|---|
| Time of day | | Seizures were 'due' (regular interval) | |
| Missed / late medication | | Medication change | |
| Missed sleep | | Missed meal | |
| Exercise | | Temperature (too hot / cold) | |
| Sensory (Loud sounds / flashing lights etc.) | | Specific food. Please note: | |
| Other medication, treatments or supplements. Please note: | | Stressful event. Please describe: | |
| Other: | | Other: | |

# *Seizure Log*

Date: _____   Time: _____   Duration: _____

Location: _____

Seizure Type: _____

If this was a cluster how many seizures? _____

Was your dog: Asleep ☐   Awake ☐   Waking from sleep ☐

What happened during the seizure?
_____
_____
_____

What was happening around the time the seizure occurred?
_____
_____
_____

Was there an Aura or warning?  Yes ☐   No ☐   Describe: _____
_____
_____

Rescue medication if given: _____

Taken to vet? Yes ☐   No ☐   Detail: _____

How long did your dog take to recover? _____

Notes:
_____
_____
_____
_____
_____

# *Seizure Log*

| What Happened During the Seizure? | | | |
|---|---|---|---|
| The seizures started with the head | | The seizure started with the limbs | |
| The seizures started on the left / right | | My dog fell down | |
| Stiff body | | Floppy body | |
| Leg paddling | | Shaking | |
| Frothing / drooling | | Chewing movements | |
| Urination | | Defecation | |
| Weakness or twitching in one part of body | | Twitching on one side of face | |
| My dog could see | | My dog could hear | |
| Other: | | Other: | |

| What Happened After the Seizure? | | | |
|---|---|---|---|
| Wobbly | | Weakness in the limbs | |
| Blindness | | Sniffing | |
| Pacing | | Disorientated | |
| Sleepy / tired | | Clingy | |
| Behaviour change: Aggressive / Fearful | | Staring into space / standing in corners | |
| Other: | | Other: | |

| Possible Triggers | | | |
|---|---|---|---|
| Time of day | | Seizures were 'due' (regular interval) | |
| Missed / late medication | | Medication change | |
| Missed sleep | | Missed meal | |
| Exercise | | Temperature (too hot / cold) | |
| Sensory (Loud sounds / flashing lights etc.) | | Specific food. Please note: | |
| Other medication, treatments or supplements. Please note: | | Stressful event. Please describe: | |
| Other: | | Other: | |

# *Seizure Log*

Date: _____ Time: _____ Duration: _____

Location: _____

Seizure Type: _____

If this was a cluster how many seizures? _____

Was your dog: Asleep ☐  Awake ☐  Waking from sleep ☐

What happened during the seizure? _____

_____

_____

_____

What was happening around the time the seizure occurred?

_____

_____

_____

Was there an Aura or warning?  Yes ☐  No ☐  Describe: _____

_____

_____

Rescue medication if given: _____

Taken to vet? Yes ☐  No ☐  Detail: _____

How long did your dog take to recover? _____

Notes: _____

_____

_____

_____

_____

_____

# *Seizure Log*

| What Happened During the Seizure? | | | |
|---|---|---|---|
| The seizures started with the head | | The seizure started with the limbs | |
| The seizures started on the left / right | | My dog fell down | |
| Stiff body | | Floppy body | |
| Leg paddling | | Shaking | |
| Frothing / drooling | | Chewing movements | |
| Urination | | Defecation | |
| Weakness or twitching in one part of body | | Twitching on one side of face | |
| My dog could see | | My dog could hear | |
| Other: | | Other: | |

| What Happened After the Seizure? | | | |
|---|---|---|---|
| Wobbly | | Weakness in the limbs | |
| Blindness | | Sniffing | |
| Pacing | | Disorientated | |
| Sleepy / tired | | Clingy | |
| Behaviour change: Aggressive / Fearful | | Staring into space / standing in corners | |
| Other: | | Other: | |

| Possible Triggers | | | |
|---|---|---|---|
| Time of day | | Seizures were 'due' (regular interval) | |
| Missed / late medication | | Medication change | |
| Missed sleep | | Missed meal | |
| Exercise | | Temperature (too hot / cold) | |
| Sensory (Loud sounds / flashing lights etc.) | | Specific food. Please note: | |
| Other medication, treatments or supplements. Please note: | | Stressful event. Please describe: | |
| Other: | | Other: | |

# *Seizure Log*

Date: _____  Time: _____  Duration: _____

Location: _____

Seizure Type: _____

If this was a cluster how many seizures? _____

Was your dog: Asleep ☐  Awake ☐  Waking from sleep ☐

What happened during the seizure? _____

_____

_____

What was happening around the time the seizure occurred? _____

_____

_____

Was there an Aura or warning?  Yes ☐  No ☐  Describe: _____

_____

_____

Rescue medication if given: _____

Taken to vet? Yes ☐  No ☐  Detail: _____

How long did your dog take to recover? _____

Notes: _____

_____

_____

_____

_____

_____

# *Seizure Log*

| What Happened During the Seizure? | | | |
|---|---|---|---|
| The seizures started with the head | | The seizure started with the limbs | |
| The seizures started on the left / right | | My dog fell down | |
| Stiff body | | Floppy body | |
| Leg paddling | | Shaking | |
| Frothing / drooling | | Chewing movements | |
| Urination | | Defecation | |
| Weakness or twitching in one part of body | | Twitching on one side of face | |
| My dog could see | | My dog could hear | |
| Other: | | Other: | |

| What Happened After the Seizure? | | | |
|---|---|---|---|
| Wobbly | | Weakness in the limbs | |
| Blindness | | Sniffing | |
| Pacing | | Disorientated | |
| Sleepy / tired | | Clingy | |
| Behaviour change: Aggressive / Fearful | | Staring into space / standing in corners | |
| Other: | | Other: | |

| Possible Triggers | | | |
|---|---|---|---|
| Time of day | | Seizures were 'due' (regular interval) | |
| Missed / late medication | | Medication change | |
| Missed sleep | | Missed meal | |
| Exercise | | Temperature (too hot / cold) | |
| Sensory (Loud sounds / flashing lights etc.) | | Specific food. Please note: | |
| Other medication, treatments or supplements. Please note: | | Stressful event. Please describe: | |
| Other: | | Other: | |

# *Seizure Log*

Date: _____     Time: _____     Duration: _____

Location: _____

Seizure Type: _____

If this was a cluster how many seizures? _____

Was your dog: Asleep ☐  Awake ☐  Waking from sleep ☐

What happened during the seizure? _____

_____

_____

_____

What was happening around the time the seizure occurred?

_____

_____

_____

Was there an Aura or warning?  Yes ☐  No ☐  Describe: _____

_____

_____

Rescue medication if given: _____

Taken to vet? Yes ☐  No ☐  Detail: _____

How long did your dog take to recover? _____

Notes: _____

_____

_____

_____

_____

_____

# Seizure Log

| What Happened During the Seizure? | | | |
|---|---|---|---|
| The seizures started with the head | | The seizure started with the limbs | |
| The seizures started on the left / right | | My dog fell down | |
| Stiff body | | Floppy body | |
| Leg paddling | | Shaking | |
| Frothing / drooling | | Chewing movements | |
| Urination | | Defecation | |
| Weakness or twitching in one part of body | | Twitching on one side of face | |
| My dog could see | | My dog could hear | |
| Other: | | Other: | |

| What Happened After the Seizure? | | | |
|---|---|---|---|
| Wobbly | | Weakness in the limbs | |
| Blindness | | Sniffing | |
| Pacing | | Disorientated | |
| Sleepy / tired | | Clingy | |
| Behaviour change: Aggressive / Fearful | | Staring into space / standing in corners | |
| Other: | | Other: | |

| Possible Triggers | | | |
|---|---|---|---|
| Time of day | | Seizures were 'due' (regular interval) | |
| Missed / late medication | | Medication change | |
| Missed sleep | | Missed meal | |
| Exercise | | Temperature (too hot / cold) | |
| Sensory (Loud sounds / flashing lights etc.) | | Specific food. Please note: | |
| Other medication, treatments or supplements. Please note: | | Stressful event. Please describe: | |
| Other: | | Other: | |

# *Seizure Log*

Date: _____ | Time: _____ | Duration: _____

Location: _____

Seizure Type: _____

If this was a cluster how many seizures? _____

Was your dog: Asleep ☐  Awake ☐  Waking from sleep ☐

What happened during the seizure? _____

_____

_____

_____

What was happening around the time the seizure occurred? _____

_____

_____

Was there an Aura or warning?  Yes ☐  No ☐  Describe: _____

_____

_____

Rescue medication if given: _____

Taken to vet? Yes ☐  No ☐  Detail: _____

How long did your dog take to recover? _____

Notes: _____

_____

_____

_____

_____

_____

# *Seizure Log*

| What Happened During the Seizure? | | | |
|---|---|---|---|
| The seizures started with the head | | The seizure started with the limbs | |
| The seizures started on the left / right | | My dog fell down | |
| Stiff body | | Floppy body | |
| Leg paddling | | Shaking | |
| Frothing / drooling | | Chewing movements | |
| Urination | | Defecation | |
| Weakness or twitching in one part of body | | Twitching on one side of face | |
| My dog could see | | My dog could hear | |
| Other: | | Other: | |

| What Happened After the Seizure? | | | |
|---|---|---|---|
| Wobbly | | Weakness in the limbs | |
| Blindness | | Sniffing | |
| Pacing | | Disorientated | |
| Sleepy / tired | | Clingy | |
| Behaviour change: Aggressive / Fearful | | Staring into space / standing in corners | |
| Other: | | Other: | |

| Possible Triggers | | | |
|---|---|---|---|
| Time of day | | Seizures were 'due' (regular interval) | |
| Missed / late medication | | Medication change | |
| Missed sleep | | Missed meal | |
| Exercise | | Temperature (too hot / cold) | |
| Sensory (Loud sounds / flashing lights etc.) | | Specific food. Please note: | |
| Other medication, treatments or supplements. Please note: | | Stressful event. Please describe: | |
| Other: | | Other: | |

# *Seizure Log*

Date: _____    Time: _____    Duration: _____

Location: _____

Seizure Type: _____

If this was a cluster how many seizures? _____

Was your dog: Asleep ☐  Awake ☐  Waking from sleep ☐

What happened during the seizure? _____

_____

_____

What was happening around the time the seizure occurred? _____

_____

_____

Was there an Aura or warning?  Yes ☐  No ☐  Describe: _____

_____

_____

Rescue medication if given: _____

Taken to vet? Yes ☐  No ☐  Detail: _____

How long did your dog take to recover? _____

Notes: _____

_____

_____

_____

_____

_____

# *Seizure Log*

| What Happened During the Seizure? | | | |
|---|---|---|---|
| The seizures started with the head | | The seizure started with the limbs | |
| The seizures started on the left / right | | My dog fell down | |
| Stiff body | | Floppy body | |
| Leg paddling | | Shaking | |
| Frothing / drooling | | Chewing movements | |
| Urination | | Defecation | |
| Weakness or twitching in one part of body | | Twitching on one side of face | |
| My dog could see | | My dog could hear | |
| Other: | | Other: | |

| What Happened After the Seizure? | | | |
|---|---|---|---|
| Wobbly | | Weakness in the limbs | |
| Blindness | | Sniffing | |
| Pacing | | Disorientated | |
| Sleepy / tired | | Clingy | |
| Behaviour change: Aggressive / Fearful | | Staring into space / standing in corners | |
| Other: | | Other: | |

| Possible Triggers | | | |
|---|---|---|---|
| Time of day | | Seizures were 'due' (regular interval) | |
| Missed / late medication | | Medication change | |
| Missed sleep | | Missed meal | |
| Exercise | | Temperature (too hot / cold) | |
| Sensory (Loud sounds / flashing lights etc.) | | Specific food. Please note: | |
| Other medication, treatments or supplements. Please note: | | Stressful event. Please describe: | |
| Other: | | Other: | |

# *Seizure Log*

Date: _____  Time: _____  Duration: _____

Location: _____

Seizure Type: _____

If this was a cluster how many seizures? _____

Was your dog: Asleep ☐  Awake ☐  Waking from sleep ☐

What happened during the seizure? _____

_____

_____

What was happening around the time the seizure occurred? _____

_____

_____

Was there an Aura or warning?  Yes ☐  No ☐  Describe: _____

_____

Rescue medication if given: _____

Taken to vet? Yes ☐  No ☐  Detail: _____

How long did your dog take to recover? _____

Notes: _____

_____

_____

_____

_____

_____

# *Seizure Log*

| What Happened During the Seizure? | | | |
|---|---|---|---|
| The seizures started with the head | | The seizure started with the limbs | |
| The seizures started on the left / right | | My dog fell down | |
| Stiff body | | Floppy body | |
| Leg paddling | | Shaking | |
| Frothing / drooling | | Chewing movements | |
| Urination | | Defecation | |
| Weakness or twitching in one part of body | | Twitching on one side of face | |
| My dog could see | | My dog could hear | |
| Other: | | Other: | |

| What Happened After the Seizure? | | | |
|---|---|---|---|
| Wobbly | | Weakness in the limbs | |
| Blindness | | Sniffing | |
| Pacing | | Disorientated | |
| Sleepy / tired | | Clingy | |
| Behaviour change: Aggressive / Fearful | | Staring into space / standing in corners | |
| Other: | | Other: | |

| Possible Triggers | | | |
|---|---|---|---|
| Time of day | | Seizures were 'due' (regular interval) | |
| Missed / late medication | | Medication change | |
| Missed sleep | | Missed meal | |
| Exercise | | Temperature (too hot / cold) | |
| Sensory (Loud sounds / flashing lights etc.) | | Specific food. Please note: | |
| Other medication, treatments or supplements. Please note: | | Stressful event. Please describe: | |
| Other: | | Other: | |

# *Seizure Log*

Date: _____  Time: _____  Duration: _____

Location: _____

Seizure Type: _____

If this was a cluster how many seizures? _____

Was your dog: Asleep ☐  Awake ☐  Waking from sleep ☐

What happened during the seizure? _____

_____

_____

What was happening around the time the seizure occurred?

_____

_____

Was there an Aura or warning?  Yes ☐  No ☐  Describe: _____

_____

Rescue medication if given: _____

Taken to vet? Yes ☐  No ☐  Detail: _____

How long did your dog take to recover? _____

Notes: _____

_____

_____

_____

_____

# Seizure Log

| What Happened During the Seizure? | | | |
|---|---|---|---|
| The seizures started with the head | | The seizure started with the limbs | |
| The seizures started on the left / right | | My dog fell down | |
| Stiff body | | Floppy body | |
| Leg paddling | | Shaking | |
| Frothing / drooling | | Chewing movements | |
| Urination | | Defecation | |
| Weakness or twitching in one part of body | | Twitching on one side of face | |
| My dog could see | | My dog could hear | |
| Other: | | Other: | |

| What Happened After the Seizure? | | | |
|---|---|---|---|
| Wobbly | | Weakness in the limbs | |
| Blindness | | Sniffing | |
| Pacing | | Disorientated | |
| Sleepy / tired | | Clingy | |
| Behaviour change: Aggressive / Fearful | | Staring into space / standing in corners | |
| Other: | | Other: | |

| Possible Triggers | | | |
|---|---|---|---|
| Time of day | | Seizures were 'due' (regular interval) | |
| Missed / late medication | | Medication change | |
| Missed sleep | | Missed meal | |
| Exercise | | Temperature (too hot / cold) | |
| Sensory (Loud sounds / flashing lights etc.) | | Specific food. Please note: | |
| Other medication, treatments or supplements. Please note: | | Stressful event. Please describe: | |
| Other: | | Other: | |

# *Seizure Log*

Date: _____    Time: _____    Duration: _____

Location: _____

Seizure Type: _____

If this was a cluster how many seizures? _____

Was your dog: Asleep ☐    Awake ☐    Waking from sleep ☐

What happened during the seizure?

_____

_____

What was happening around the time the seizure occurred?

_____

_____

Was there an Aura or warning?  Yes ☐    No ☐    Describe: _____

_____

Rescue medication if given: _____

Taken to vet? Yes ☐    No ☐    Detail: _____

How long did your dog take to recover? _____

Notes:

_____

_____

_____

_____

# *Seizure Log*

| What Happened During the Seizure? | | | |
|---|---|---|---|
| The seizures started with the head | | The seizure started with the limbs | |
| The seizures started on the left / right | | My dog fell down | |
| Stiff body | | Floppy body | |
| Leg paddling | | Shaking | |
| Frothing / drooling | | Chewing movements | |
| Urination | | Defecation | |
| Weakness or twitching in one part of body | | Twitching on one side of face | |
| My dog could see | | My dog could hear | |
| Other: | | Other: | |

| What Happened After the Seizure? | | | |
|---|---|---|---|
| Wobbly | | Weakness in the limbs | |
| Blindness | | Sniffing | |
| Pacing | | Disorientated | |
| Sleepy / tired | | Clingy | |
| Behaviour change: Aggressive / Fearful | | Staring into space / standing in corners | |
| Other: | | Other: | |

| Possible Triggers | | | |
|---|---|---|---|
| Time of day | | Seizures were 'due' (regular interval) | |
| Missed / late medication | | Medication change | |
| Missed sleep | | Missed meal | |
| Exercise | | Temperature (too hot / cold) | |
| Sensory (Loud sounds / flashing lights etc.) | | Specific food. Please note: | |
| Other medication, treatments or supplements. Please note: | | Stressful event. Please describe: | |
| Other: | | Other: | |

# *Seizure Log*

Date: _____ Time: _____ Duration: _____

Location: _____

Seizure Type: _____

If this was a cluster how many seizures? _____

Was your dog: Asleep ☐  Awake ☐  Waking from sleep ☐

What happened during the seizure?

_____

_____

_____

What was happening around the time the seizure occurred?

_____

_____

Was there an Aura or warning?  Yes ☐  No ☐  Describe: _____

_____

Rescue medication if given: _____

Taken to vet? Yes ☐  No ☐  Detail: _____

How long did your dog take to recover? _____

Notes:

_____

_____

_____

_____

_____

# *Seizure Log*

| What Happened During the Seizure? | | | |
|---|---|---|---|
| The seizures started with the head | | The seizure started with the limbs | |
| The seizures started on the left / right | | My dog fell down | |
| Stiff body | | Floppy body | |
| Leg paddling | | Shaking | |
| Frothing / drooling | | Chewing movements | |
| Urination | | Defecation | |
| Weakness or twitching in one part of body | | Twitching on one side of face | |
| My dog could see | | My dog could hear | |
| Other: | | Other: | |

| What Happened After the Seizure? | | | |
|---|---|---|---|
| Wobbly | | Weakness in the limbs | |
| Blindness | | Sniffing | |
| Pacing | | Disorientated | |
| Sleepy / tired | | Clingy | |
| Behaviour change: Aggressive / Fearful | | Staring into space / standing in corners | |
| Other: | | Other: | |

| Possible Triggers | | | |
|---|---|---|---|
| Time of day | | Seizures were 'due' (regular interval) | |
| Missed / late medication | | Medication change | |
| Missed sleep | | Missed meal | |
| Exercise | | Temperature (too hot / cold) | |
| Sensory (Loud sounds / flashing lights etc.) | | Specific food. Please note: | |
| Other medication, treatments or supplements. Please note: | | Stressful event. Please describe: | |
| Other: | | Other: | |

# *Seizure Log*

Date: _____     Time: _____     Duration: _____

Location: _____

Seizure Type: _____

If this was a cluster how many seizures? _____

Was your dog: Asleep ☐   Awake ☐   Waking from sleep ☐

What happened during the seizure?

_____

_____

_____

What was happening around the time the seizure occurred?

_____

_____

Was there an Aura or warning?  Yes ☐   No ☐   Describe: _____

_____

Rescue medication if given: _____

Taken to vet? Yes ☐   No ☐   Detail: _____

How long did your dog take to recover? _____

Notes:

_____

_____

_____

_____

_____

# *Seizure Log*

| What Happened During the Seizure? | | | |
|---|---|---|---|
| The seizures started with the head | | The seizure started with the limbs | |
| The seizures started on the left / right | | My dog fell down | |
| Stiff body | | Floppy body | |
| Leg paddling | | Shaking | |
| Frothing / drooling | | Chewing movements | |
| Urination | | Defecation | |
| Weakness or twitching in one part of body | | Twitching on one side of face | |
| My dog could see | | My dog could hear | |
| Other: | | Other: | |

| What Happened After the Seizure? | | | |
|---|---|---|---|
| Wobbly | | Weakness in the limbs | |
| Blindness | | Sniffing | |
| Pacing | | Disorientated | |
| Sleepy / tired | | Clingy | |
| Behaviour change: Aggressive / Fearful | | Staring into space / standing in corners | |
| Other: | | Other: | |

| Possible Triggers | | | |
|---|---|---|---|
| Time of day | | Seizures were 'due' (regular interval) | |
| Missed / late medication | | Medication change | |
| Missed sleep | | Missed meal | |
| Exercise | | Temperature (too hot / cold) | |
| Sensory (Loud sounds / flashing lights etc.) | | Specific food. Please note: | |
| Other medication, treatments or supplements. Please note: | | Stressful event. Please describe: | |
| Other: | | Other: | |

# *Seizure Log*

Date: _____  Time: _____  Duration: _____

Location: _____

Seizure Type: _____

If this was a cluster how many seizures? _____

Was your dog: Asleep ☐  Awake ☐  Waking from sleep ☐

What happened during the seizure? _____

_____

_____

What was happening around the time the seizure occurred?

_____

_____

Was there an Aura or warning?  Yes ☐  No ☐  Describe: _____

_____

Rescue medication if given: _____

Taken to vet? Yes ☐  No ☐  Detail: _____

How long did your dog take to recover? _____

Notes: _____

_____

_____

_____

_____

# Seizure Log

| What Happened During the Seizure? | | | |
|---|---|---|---|
| The seizures started with the head | | The seizure started with the limbs | |
| The seizures started on the left / right | | My dog fell down | |
| Stiff body | | Floppy body | |
| Leg paddling | | Shaking | |
| Frothing / drooling | | Chewing movements | |
| Urination | | Defecation | |
| Weakness or twitching in one part of body | | Twitching on one side of face | |
| My dog could see | | My dog could hear | |
| Other: | | Other: | |

| What Happened After the Seizure? | | | |
|---|---|---|---|
| Wobbly | | Weakness in the limbs | |
| Blindness | | Sniffing | |
| Pacing | | Disorientated | |
| Sleepy / tired | | Clingy | |
| Behaviour change: Aggressive / Fearful | | Staring into space / standing in corners | |
| Other: | | Other: | |

| Possible Triggers | | | |
|---|---|---|---|
| Time of day | | Seizures were 'due' (regular interval) | |
| Missed / late medication | | Medication change | |
| Missed sleep | | Missed meal | |
| Exercise | | Temperature (too hot / cold) | |
| Sensory (Loud sounds / flashing lights etc.) | | Specific food. Please note: | |
| Other medication, treatments or supplements. Please note: | | Stressful event. Please describe: | |
| Other: | | Other: | |

# *Seizure Log*

Date: _____    Time: _____    Duration: _____

Location: _____

Seizure Type: _____

If this was a cluster how many seizures? _____

Was your dog: Asleep ☐    Awake ☐    Waking from sleep ☐

What happened during the seizure?

_____

_____

_____

What was happening around the time the seizure occurred?

_____

_____

Was there an Aura or warning?  Yes ☐  No ☐  Describe: _____

_____

Rescue medication if given: _____

Taken to vet? Yes ☐  No ☐  Detail: _____

How long did your dog take to recover? _____

Notes:

_____

_____

_____

_____

# Seizure Log

| What Happened During the Seizure? | | |
|---|---|---|
| The seizures started with the head | The seizure started with the limbs | |
| The seizures started on the left / right | My dog fell down | |
| Stiff body | Floppy body | |
| Leg paddling | Shaking | |
| Frothing / drooling | Chewing movements | |
| Urination | Defecation | |
| Weakness or twitching in one part of body | Twitching on one side of face | |
| My dog could see | My dog could hear | |
| Other: | Other: | |

| What Happened After the Seizure? | | |
|---|---|---|
| Wobbly | Weakness in the limbs | |
| Blindness | Sniffing | |
| Pacing | Disorientated | |
| Sleepy / tired | Clingy | |
| Behaviour change: Aggressive / Fearful | Staring into space / standing in corners | |
| Other: | Other: | |

| Possible Triggers | | |
|---|---|---|
| Time of day | Seizures were 'due' (regular interval) | |
| Missed / late medication | Medication change | |
| Missed sleep | Missed meal | |
| Exercise | Temperature (too hot / cold) | |
| Sensory (Loud sounds / flashing lights etc.) | Specific food. Please note: | |
| Other medication, treatments or supplements. Please note: | Stressful event. Please describe: | |
| Other: | Other: | |

103

# *Seizure Log*

Date: _____    Time: _____    Duration: _____

Location: _____

Seizure Type: _____

If this was a cluster how many seizures? _____

Was your dog: Asleep ☐  Awake ☐  Waking from sleep ☐

What happened during the seizure? _____

_____

_____

What was happening around the time the seizure occurred?

_____

_____

Was there an Aura or warning?  Yes ☐  No ☐  Describe: _____

_____

_____

Rescue medication if given: _____

Taken to vet? Yes ☐  No ☐  Detail: _____

How long did your dog take to recover? _____

Notes: _____

_____

_____

_____

_____

_____

# *Seizure Log*

| What Happened During the Seizure? | | | |
|---|---|---|---|
| The seizures started with the head | | The seizure started with the limbs | |
| The seizures started on the left / right | | My dog fell down | |
| Stiff body | | Floppy body | |
| Leg paddling | | Shaking | |
| Frothing / drooling | | Chewing movements | |
| Urination | | Defecation | |
| Weakness or twitching in one part of body | | Twitching on one side of face | |
| My dog could see | | My dog could hear | |
| Other: | | Other: | |

| What Happened After the Seizure? | | | |
|---|---|---|---|
| Wobbly | | Weakness in the limbs | |
| Blindness | | Sniffing | |
| Pacing | | Disorientated | |
| Sleepy / tired | | Clingy | |
| Behaviour change: Aggressive / Fearful | | Staring into space / standing in corners | |
| Other: | | Other: | |

| Possible Triggers | | | |
|---|---|---|---|
| Time of day | | Seizures were 'due' (regular interval) | |
| Missed / late medication | | Medication change | |
| Missed sleep | | Missed meal | |
| Exercise | | Temperature (too hot / cold) | |
| Sensory (Loud sounds / flashing lights etc.) | | Specific food. Please note: | |
| Other medication, treatments or supplements. Please note: | | Stressful event. Please describe: | |
| Other: | | Other: | |

# *Seizure Log*

Date: _____     Time: _____     Duration: _____

Location: _____

Seizure Type: _____

If this was a cluster how many seizures? _____

Was your dog: Asleep ☐     Awake ☐     Waking from sleep ☐

What happened during the seizure? _____
_____
_____
_____

What was happening around the time the seizure occurred?
_____
_____
_____

Was there an Aura or warning?  Yes ☐   No ☐   Describe: _____
_____
_____

Rescue medication if given: _____

Taken to vet? Yes ☐   No ☐   Detail: _____

How long did your dog take to recover? _____

Notes: _____
_____
_____
_____
_____
_____

# *Seizure Log*

| What Happened During the Seizure? | | | |
|---|---|---|---|
| The seizures started with the head | | The seizure started with the limbs | |
| The seizures started on the left / right | | My dog fell down | |
| Stiff body | | Floppy body | |
| Leg paddling | | Shaking | |
| Frothing / drooling | | Chewing movements | |
| Urination | | Defecation | |
| Weakness or twitching in one part of body | | Twitching on one side of face | |
| My dog could see | | My dog could hear | |
| Other: | | Other: | |

| What Happened After the Seizure? | | | |
|---|---|---|---|
| Wobbly | | Weakness in the limbs | |
| Blindness | | Sniffing | |
| Pacing | | Disorientated | |
| Sleepy / tired | | Clingy | |
| Behaviour change: Aggressive / Fearful | | Staring into space / standing in corners | |
| Other: | | Other: | |

| Possible Triggers | | | |
|---|---|---|---|
| Time of day | | Seizures were 'due' (regular interval) | |
| Missed / late medication | | Medication change | |
| Missed sleep | | Missed meal | |
| Exercise | | Temperature (too hot / cold) | |
| Sensory (Loud sounds / flashing lights etc.) | | Specific food. Please note: | |
| Other medication, treatments or supplements. Please note: | | Stressful event. Please describe: | |
| Other: | | Other: | |

# *Seizure Log*

Date: _____    Time: _____    Duration: _____

Location: _____

Seizure Type: _____

If this was a cluster how many seizures? _____

Was your dog: Asleep ☐    Awake ☐    Waking from sleep ☐

What happened during the seizure? _____

_____

_____

What was happening around the time the seizure occurred? _____

_____

_____

Was there an Aura or warning?  Yes ☐  No ☐  Describe: _____

_____

_____

Rescue medication if given: _____

Taken to vet? Yes ☐  No ☐  Detail: _____

How long did your dog take to recover? _____

Notes: _____

_____

_____

_____

_____

_____

# Seizure Log

| What Happened During the Seizure? | | | |
|---|---|---|---|
| The seizures started with the head | | The seizure started with the limbs | |
| The seizures started on the left / right | | My dog fell down | |
| Stiff body | | Floppy body | |
| Leg paddling | | Shaking | |
| Frothing / drooling | | Chewing movements | |
| Urination | | Defecation | |
| Weakness or twitching in one part of body | | Twitching on one side of face | |
| My dog could see | | My dog could hear | |
| Other: | | Other: | |

| What Happened After the Seizure? | | | |
|---|---|---|---|
| Wobbly | | Weakness in the limbs | |
| Blindness | | Sniffing | |
| Pacing | | Disorientated | |
| Sleepy / tired | | Clingy | |
| Behaviour change: Aggressive / Fearful | | Staring into space / standing in corners | |
| Other: | | Other: | |

| Possible Triggers | | | |
|---|---|---|---|
| Time of day | | Seizures were 'due' (regular interval) | |
| Missed / late medication | | Medication change | |
| Missed sleep | | Missed meal | |
| Exercise | | Temperature (too hot / cold) | |
| Sensory (Loud sounds / flashing lights etc.) | | Specific food. Please note: | |
| Other medication, treatments or supplements. Please note: | | Stressful event. Please describe: | |
| Other: | | Other: | |

# *Seizure Log*

Date: _____ Time: _____ Duration: _____

Location: _____

Seizure Type: _____

If this was a cluster how many seizures? _____

Was your dog: Asleep ☐  Awake ☐  Waking from sleep ☐

What happened during the seizure? _____

_____

_____

What was happening around the time the seizure occurred? _____

_____

_____

Was there an Aura or warning?  Yes ☐  No ☐  Describe: _____

_____

Rescue medication if given: _____

Taken to vet? Yes ☐  No ☐  Detail: _____

How long did your dog take to recover? _____

Notes: _____

_____

_____

_____

_____

_____

# *Seizure Log*

## What Happened During the Seizure?

| | | | |
|---|---|---|---|
| The seizures started with the head | | The seizure started with the limbs | |
| The seizures started on the left / right | | My dog fell down | |
| Stiff body | | Floppy body | |
| Leg paddling | | Shaking | |
| Frothing / drooling | | Chewing movements | |
| Urination | | Defecation | |
| Weakness or twitching in one part of body | | Twitching on one side of face | |
| My dog could see | | My dog could hear | |
| Other: | | Other: | |

## What Happened After the Seizure?

| | | | |
|---|---|---|---|
| Wobbly | | Weakness in the limbs | |
| Blindness | | Sniffing | |
| Pacing | | Disorientated | |
| Sleepy / tired | | Clingy | |
| Behaviour change: Aggressive / Fearful | | Staring into space / standing in corners | |
| Other: | | Other: | |

## Possible Triggers

| | | | |
|---|---|---|---|
| Time of day | | Seizures were 'due' (regular interval) | |
| Missed / late medication | | Medication change | |
| Missed sleep | | Missed meal | |
| Exercise | | Temperature (too hot / cold) | |
| Sensory (Loud sounds / flashing lights etc.) | | Specific food. Please note: | |
| Other medication, treatments or supplements. Please note: | | Stressful event. Please describe: | |
| Other: | | Other: | |

# *Seizure Log*

Date: _____  Time: _____  Duration: _____

Location: _____

Seizure Type: _____

If this was a cluster how many seizures? _____

Was your dog: Asleep ☐  Awake ☐  Waking from sleep ☐

What happened during the seizure?

_____

_____

_____

What was happening around the time the seizure occurred?

_____

_____

_____

Was there an Aura or warning?  Yes ☐  No ☐  Describe: _____

_____

_____

Rescue medication if given: _____

Taken to vet? Yes ☐  No ☐  Detail: _____

How long did your dog take to recover? _____

Notes:

_____

_____

_____

_____

_____

_____

# *Seizure Log*

| What Happened During the Seizure? | | | |
|---|---|---|---|
| The seizures started with the head | | The seizure started with the limbs | |
| The seizures started on the left / right | | My dog fell down | |
| Stiff body | | Floppy body | |
| Leg paddling | | Shaking | |
| Frothing / drooling | | Chewing movements | |
| Urination | | Defecation | |
| Weakness or twitching in one part of body | | Twitching on one side of face | |
| My dog could see | | My dog could hear | |
| Other: | | Other: | |

| What Happened After the Seizure? | | | |
|---|---|---|---|
| Wobbly | | Weakness in the limbs | |
| Blindness | | Sniffing | |
| Pacing | | Disorientated | |
| Sleepy / tired | | Clingy | |
| Behaviour change: Aggressive / Fearful | | Staring into space / standing in corners | |
| Other: | | Other: | |

| Possible Triggers | | | |
|---|---|---|---|
| Time of day | | Seizures were 'due' (regular interval) | |
| Missed / late medication | | Medication change | |
| Missed sleep | | Missed meal | |
| Exercise | | Temperature (too hot / cold) | |
| Sensory (Loud sounds / flashing lights etc.) | | Specific food. Please note: | |
| Other medication, treatments or supplements. Please note: | | Stressful event. Please describe: | |
| Other: | | Other: | |

# *Seizure Log*

Date: _____    Time: _____    Duration: _____

Location: _____

Seizure Type: _____

If this was a cluster how many seizures? _____

Was your dog: Asleep ☐   Awake ☐   Waking from sleep ☐

What happened during the seizure? _____

_____

_____

_____

What was happening around the time the seizure occurred?

_____

_____

_____

Was there an Aura or warning?  Yes ☐   No ☐   Describe: _____

_____

_____

Rescue medication if given: _____

Taken to vet? Yes ☐   No ☐   Detail: _____

How long did your dog take to recover? _____

Notes: _____

_____

_____

_____

_____

_____

# Seizure Log

| What Happened During the Seizure? | | |
|---|---|---|
| The seizures started with the head | The seizure started with the limbs | |
| The seizures started on the left / right | My dog fell down | |
| Stiff body | Floppy body | |
| Leg paddling | Shaking | |
| Frothing / drooling | Chewing movements | |
| Urination | Defecation | |
| Weakness or twitching in one part of body | Twitching on one side of face | |
| My dog could see | My dog could hear | |
| Other: | Other: | |

| What Happened After the Seizure? | | |
|---|---|---|
| Wobbly | Weakness in the limbs | |
| Blindness | Sniffing | |
| Pacing | Disorientated | |
| Sleepy / tired | Clingy | |
| Behaviour change: Aggressive / Fearful | Staring into space / standing in corners | |
| Other: | Other: | |

| Possible Triggers | | |
|---|---|---|
| Time of day | Seizures were 'due' (regular interval) | |
| Missed / late medication | Medication change | |
| Missed sleep | Missed meal | |
| Exercise | Temperature (too hot / cold) | |
| Sensory (Loud sounds / flashing lights etc.) | Specific food. Please note: | |
| Other medication, treatments or supplements. Please note: | Stressful event. Please describe: | |
| Other: | Other: | |

# *Seizure Log*

Date: _____    Time: _____    Duration: _____

Location: _____

Seizure Type: _____

If this was a cluster how many seizures? _____

Was your dog: Asleep ☐  Awake ☐  Waking from sleep ☐

What happened during the seizure? _____

_____

_____

What was happening around the time the seizure occurred?

_____

_____

Was there an Aura or warning?  Yes ☐  No ☐  Describe: _____

_____

Rescue medication if given: _____

Taken to vet? Yes ☐  No ☐  Detail: _____

How long did your dog take to recover? _____

Notes:

_____

_____

_____

_____

_____

# *Seizure Log*

| What Happened During the Seizure? | | |
|---|---|---|
| The seizures started with the head | The seizure started with the limbs | |
| The seizures started on the left / right | My dog fell down | |
| Stiff body | Floppy body | |
| Leg paddling | Shaking | |
| Frothing / drooling | Chewing movements | |
| Urination | Defecation | |
| Weakness or twitching in one part of body | Twitching on one side of face | |
| My dog could see | My dog could hear | |
| Other: | Other: | |

| What Happened After the Seizure? | | |
|---|---|---|
| Wobbly | Weakness in the limbs | |
| Blindness | Sniffing | |
| Pacing | Disorientated | |
| Sleepy / tired | Clingy | |
| Behaviour change: Aggressive / Fearful | Staring into space / standing in corners | |
| Other: | Other: | |

| Possible Triggers | | |
|---|---|---|
| Time of day | Seizures were 'due' (regular interval) | |
| Missed / late medication | Medication change | |
| Missed sleep | Missed meal | |
| Exercise | Temperature (too hot / cold) | |
| Sensory (Loud sounds / flashing lights etc.) | Specific food. Please note: | |
| Other medication, treatments or supplements. Please note: | Stressful event. Please describe: | |
| Other: | Other: | |

# Seizure Log

Date: _____  Time: _____  Duration: _____

Location: _____

Seizure Type: _____

If this was a cluster how many seizures? _____

Was your dog: Asleep ☐  Awake ☐  Waking from sleep ☐

What happened during the seizure? _____

_____

_____

_____

What was happening around the time the seizure occurred?

_____

_____

_____

Was there an Aura or warning?  Yes ☐  No ☐  Describe: _____

_____

_____

Rescue medication if given: _____

Taken to vet? Yes ☐  No ☐  Detail: _____

How long did your dog take to recover? _____

Notes: _____

_____

_____

_____

_____

_____

# Seizure Log

| What Happened During the Seizure? | | |
|---|---|---|
| The seizures started with the head | The seizure started with the limbs | |
| The seizures started on the left / right | My dog fell down | |
| Stiff body | Floppy body | |
| Leg paddling | Shaking | |
| Frothing / drooling | Chewing movements | |
| Urination | Defecation | |
| Weakness or twitching in one part of body | Twitching on one side of face | |
| My dog could see | My dog could hear | |
| Other: | Other: | |

| What Happened After the Seizure? | | |
|---|---|---|
| Wobbly | Weakness in the limbs | |
| Blindness | Sniffing | |
| Pacing | Disorientated | |
| Sleepy / tired | Clingy | |
| Behaviour change: Aggressive / Fearful | Staring into space / standing in corners | |
| Other: | Other: | |

| Possible Triggers | | |
|---|---|---|
| Time of day | Seizures were 'due' (regular interval) | |
| Missed / late medication | Medication change | |
| Missed sleep | Missed meal | |
| Exercise | Temperature (too hot / cold) | |
| Sensory (Loud sounds / flashing lights etc.) | Specific food. Please note: | |
| Other medication, treatments or supplements. Please note: | Stressful event. Please describe: | |
| Other: | Other: | |

119

# Seizure Log

Date: _____     Time: _____     Duration: _____

Location: _____

Seizure Type: _____

If this was a cluster how many seizures? _____

Was your dog: Asleep ☐  Awake ☐  Waking from sleep ☐

What happened during the seizure? _____

_____

_____

What was happening around the time the seizure occurred?

_____

_____

Was there an Aura or warning?  Yes ☐  No ☐  Describe: _____

_____

Rescue medication if given: _____

Taken to vet? Yes ☐  No ☐  Detail: _____

How long did your dog take to recover? _____

Notes: _____

_____

_____

_____

_____

_____

# *Seizure Log*

| What Happened During the Seizure? | | |
|---|---|---|
| The seizures started with the head | The seizure started with the limbs | |
| The seizures started on the left / right | My dog fell down | |
| Stiff body | Floppy body | |
| Leg paddling | Shaking | |
| Frothing / drooling | Chewing movements | |
| Urination | Defecation | |
| Weakness or twitching in one part of body | Twitching on one side of face | |
| My dog could see | My dog could hear | |
| Other: | Other: | |

| What Happened After the Seizure? | | |
|---|---|---|
| Wobbly | Weakness in the limbs | |
| Blindness | Sniffing | |
| Pacing | Disorientated | |
| Sleepy / tired | Clingy | |
| Behaviour change: Aggressive / Fearful | Staring into space / standing in corners | |
| Other: | Other: | |

| Possible Triggers | | |
|---|---|---|
| Time of day | Seizures were 'due' (regular interval) | |
| Missed / late medication | Medication change | |
| Missed sleep | Missed meal | |
| Exercise | Temperature (too hot / cold) | |
| Sensory (Loud sounds / flashing lights etc.) | Specific food. Please note: | |
| Other medication, treatments or supplements. Please note: | Stressful event. Please describe: | |
| Other: | Other: | |

121

# *Seizure Log*

Date: _____   Time: _____   Duration: _____

Location: _____

Seizure Type: _____

If this was a cluster how many seizures? _____

Was your dog: Asleep ☐   Awake ☐   Waking from sleep ☐

What happened during the seizure? _____

_____

_____

What was happening around the time the seizure occurred?

_____

_____

Was there an Aura or warning?  Yes ☐   No ☐   Describe: _____

_____

Rescue medication if given: _____

Taken to vet? Yes ☐   No ☐   Detail: _____

How long did your dog take to recover? _____

Notes: _____

_____

_____

_____

_____

_____

# *Seizure Log*

| What Happened During the Seizure? | | |
|---|---|---|
| The seizures started with the head | The seizure started with the limbs | |
| The seizures started on the left / right | My dog fell down | |
| Stiff body | Floppy body | |
| Leg paddling | Shaking | |
| Frothing / drooling | Chewing movements | |
| Urination | Defecation | |
| Weakness or twitching in one part of body | Twitching on one side of face | |
| My dog could see | My dog could hear | |
| Other: | Other: | |

| What Happened After the Seizure? | | |
|---|---|---|
| Wobbly | Weakness in the limbs | |
| Blindness | Sniffing | |
| Pacing | Disorientated | |
| Sleepy / tired | Clingy | |
| Behaviour change: Aggressive / Fearful | Staring into space / standing in corners | |
| Other: | Other: | |

| Possible Triggers | | |
|---|---|---|
| Time of day | Seizures were 'due' (regular interval) | |
| Missed / late medication | Medication change | |
| Missed sleep | Missed meal | |
| Exercise | Temperature (too hot / cold) | |
| Sensory (Loud sounds / flashing lights etc.) | Specific food. Please note: | |
| Other medication, treatments or supplements. Please note: | Stressful event. Please describe: | |
| Other: | Other: | |

123

# *Seizure Log*

Date: _____     Time: _____     Duration: _____

Location: _____

Seizure Type: _____

If this was a cluster how many seizures? _____

Was your dog: Asleep ☐   Awake ☐   Waking from sleep ☐

What happened during the seizure? _____

_____

_____

_____

What was happening around the time the seizure occurred?

_____

_____

_____

Was there an Aura or warning?  Yes ☐   No ☐   Describe: _____

_____

_____

Rescue medication if given: _____

Taken to vet? Yes ☐   No ☐   Detail: _____

How long did your dog take to recover? _____

Notes: _____

_____

_____

_____

_____

# Seizure Log

| What Happened During the Seizure? | | |
|---|---|---|
| The seizures started with the head | The seizure started with the limbs | |
| The seizures started on the left / right | My dog fell down | |
| Stiff body | Floppy body | |
| Leg paddling | Shaking | |
| Frothing / drooling | Chewing movements | |
| Urination | Defecation | |
| Weakness or twitching in one part of body | Twitching on one side of face | |
| My dog could see | My dog could hear | |
| Other: | Other: | |

| What Happened After the Seizure? | | |
|---|---|---|
| Wobbly | Weakness in the limbs | |
| Blindness | Sniffing | |
| Pacing | Disorientated | |
| Sleepy / tired | Clingy | |
| Behaviour change: Aggressive / Fearful | Staring into space / standing in corners | |
| Other: | Other: | |

| Possible Triggers | | |
|---|---|---|
| Time of day | Seizures were 'due' (regular interval) | |
| Missed / late medication | Medication change | |
| Missed sleep | Missed meal | |
| Exercise | Temperature (too hot / cold) | |
| Sensory (Loud sounds / flashing lights etc.) | Specific food. Please note: | |
| Other medication, treatments or supplements. Please note: | Stressful event. Please describe: | |
| Other: | Other: | |

# *Seizure Log*

Date: _____ Time: _____ Duration: _____

Location: _____

Seizure Type: _____

If this was a cluster how many seizures? _____

Was your dog: Asleep ☐ Awake ☐ Waking from sleep ☐

What happened during the seizure? _____

_____

_____

_____

What was happening around the time the seizure occurred?

_____

_____

_____

Was there an Aura or warning? Yes ☐ No ☐ Describe: _____

_____

_____

Rescue medication if given: _____

Taken to vet? Yes ☐ No ☐ Detail: _____

How long did your dog take to recover? _____

Notes: _____

_____

_____

_____

_____

_____

# *Seizure Log*

| What Happened During the Seizure? | | | |
|---|---|---|---|
| The seizures started with the head | | The seizure started with the limbs | |
| The seizures started on the left / right | | My dog fell down | |
| Stiff body | | Floppy body | |
| Leg paddling | | Shaking | |
| Frothing / drooling | | Chewing movements | |
| Urination | | Defecation | |
| Weakness or twitching in one part of body | | Twitching on one side of face | |
| My dog could see | | My dog could hear | |
| Other: | | Other: | |

| What Happened After the Seizure? | | | |
|---|---|---|---|
| Wobbly | | Weakness in the limbs | |
| Blindness | | Sniffing | |
| Pacing | | Disorientated | |
| Sleepy / tired | | Clingy | |
| Behaviour change: Aggressive / Fearful | | Staring into space / standing in corners | |
| Other: | | Other: | |

| Possible Triggers | | | |
|---|---|---|---|
| Time of day | | Seizures were 'due' (regular interval) | |
| Missed / late medication | | Medication change | |
| Missed sleep | | Missed meal | |
| Exercise | | Temperature (too hot / cold) | |
| Sensory (Loud sounds / flashing lights etc.) | | Specific food. Please note: | |
| Other medication, treatments or supplements. Please note: | | Stressful event. Please describe: | |
| Other: | | Other: | |

# *Seizure Log*

Date: _____    Time: _____    Duration: _____

Location: _____

Seizure Type: _____

If this was a cluster how many seizures? _____

Was your dog: Asleep ☐  Awake ☐  Waking from sleep ☐

What happened during the seizure?

_____

_____

What was happening around the time the seizure occurred?

_____

_____

Was there an Aura or warning?  Yes ☐  No ☐  Describe: _____

_____

Rescue medication if given: _____

Taken to vet? Yes ☐  No ☐  Detail: _____

How long did your dog take to recover?

_____

Notes:

_____

_____

_____

_____

_____

# *Seizure Log*

| What Happened During the Seizure? | | | |
|---|---|---|---|
| The seizures started with the head | | The seizure started with the limbs | |
| The seizures started on the left / right | | My dog fell down | |
| Stiff body | | Floppy body | |
| Leg paddling | | Shaking | |
| Frothing / drooling | | Chewing movements | |
| Urination | | Defecation | |
| Weakness or twitching in one part of body | | Twitching on one side of face | |
| My dog could see | | My dog could hear | |
| Other: | | Other: | |

| What Happened After the Seizure? | | | |
|---|---|---|---|
| Wobbly | | Weakness in the limbs | |
| Blindness | | Sniffing | |
| Pacing | | Disorientated | |
| Sleepy / tired | | Clingy | |
| Behaviour change: Aggressive / Fearful | | Staring into space / standing in corners | |
| Other: | | Other: | |

| Possible Triggers | | | |
|---|---|---|---|
| Time of day | | Seizures were 'due' (regular interval) | |
| Missed / late medication | | Medication change | |
| Missed sleep | | Missed meal | |
| Exercise | | Temperature (too hot / cold) | |
| Sensory (Loud sounds / flashing lights etc.) | | Specific food. Please note: | |
| Other medication, treatments or supplements. Please note: | | Stressful event. Please describe: | |
| Other: | | Other: | |

## *Seizure Log*

Date: _____  Time: _____  Duration: _____

Location: _____

Seizure Type: _____

If this was a cluster how many seizures? _____

Was your dog: Asleep ☐  Awake ☐  Waking from sleep ☐

What happened during the seizure? _____

_____

_____

_____

What was happening around the time the seizure occurred?

_____

_____

_____

Was there an Aura or warning?  Yes ☐  No ☐  Describe: _____

_____

_____

Rescue medication if given: _____

Taken to vet? Yes ☐  No ☐  Detail: _____

How long did your dog take to recover? _____

_____

Notes: _____

_____

_____

_____

_____

_____

_____

# *Seizure Log*

| What Happened During the Seizure? | | | |
|---|---|---|---|
| The seizures started with the head | | The seizure started with the limbs | |
| The seizures started on the left / right | | My dog fell down | |
| Stiff body | | Floppy body | |
| Leg paddling | | Shaking | |
| Frothing / drooling | | Chewing movements | |
| Urination | | Defecation | |
| Weakness or twitching in one part of body | | Twitching on one side of face | |
| My dog could see | | My dog could hear | |
| Other: | | Other: | |

| What Happened After the Seizure? | | | |
|---|---|---|---|
| Wobbly | | Weakness in the limbs | |
| Blindness | | Sniffing | |
| Pacing | | Disorientated | |
| Sleepy / tired | | Clingy | |
| Behaviour change: Aggressive / Fearful | | Staring into space / standing in corners | |
| Other: | | Other: | |

| Possible Triggers | | | |
|---|---|---|---|
| Time of day | | Seizures were 'due' (regular interval) | |
| Missed / late medication | | Medication change | |
| Missed sleep | | Missed meal | |
| Exercise | | Temperature (too hot / cold) | |
| Sensory (Loud sounds / flashing lights etc.) | | Specific food. Please note: | |
| Other medication, treatments or supplements. Please note: | | Stressful event. Please describe: | |
| Other: | | Other: | |

# *Seizure Log*

Date: _____  Time: _____  Duration: _____

Location: _____

Seizure Type: _____

If this was a cluster how many seizures? _____

Was your dog: Asleep ☐  Awake ☐  Waking from sleep ☐

What happened during the seizure? _____

_____

_____

What was happening around the time the seizure occurred?

_____

_____

Was there an Aura or warning?  Yes ☐  No ☐  Describe: _____

_____

Rescue medication if given: _____

Taken to vet? Yes ☐  No ☐  Detail: _____

How long did your dog take to recover? _____

Notes: _____

_____

_____

_____

_____

# Seizure Log

| What Happened During the Seizure? | | |
|---|---|---|
| The seizures started with the head | The seizure started with the limbs | |
| The seizures started on the left / right | My dog fell down | |
| Stiff body | Floppy body | |
| Leg paddling | Shaking | |
| Frothing / drooling | Chewing movements | |
| Urination | Defecation | |
| Weakness or twitching in one part of body | Twitching on one side of face | |
| My dog could see | My dog could hear | |
| Other: | Other: | |

| What Happened After the Seizure? | | |
|---|---|---|
| Wobbly | Weakness in the limbs | |
| Blindness | Sniffing | |
| Pacing | Disorientated | |
| Sleepy / tired | Clingy | |
| Behaviour change: Aggressive / Fearful | Staring into space / standing in corners | |
| Other: | Other: | |

| Possible Triggers | | |
|---|---|---|
| Time of day | Seizures were 'due' (regular interval) | |
| Missed / late medication | Medication change | |
| Missed sleep | Missed meal | |
| Exercise | Temperature (too hot / cold) | |
| Sensory (Loud sounds / flashing lights etc.) | Specific food. Please note: | |
| Other medication, treatments or supplements. Please note: | Stressful event. Please describe: | |
| Other: | Other: | |

133

# *Seizure Log*

Date: _____ Time: _____ Duration: _____

Location: _____

Seizure Type: _____

If this was a cluster how many seizures? _____

Was your dog: Asleep ☐ Awake ☐ Waking from sleep ☐

What happened during the seizure? _____

_____

_____

What was happening around the time the seizure occurred?

_____

_____

Was there an Aura or warning? Yes ☐ No ☐ Describe: _____

_____

Rescue medication if given: _____

Taken to vet? Yes ☐ No ☐ Detail: _____

How long did your dog take to recover? _____

Notes:

_____

_____

_____

_____

_____

# Seizure Log

| What Happened During the Seizure? | | | |
|---|---|---|---|
| The seizures started with the head | | The seizure started with the limbs | |
| The seizures started on the left / right | | My dog fell down | |
| Stiff body | | Floppy body | |
| Leg paddling | | Shaking | |
| Frothing / drooling | | Chewing movements | |
| Urination | | Defecation | |
| Weakness or twitching in one part of body | | Twitching on one side of face | |
| My dog could see | | My dog could hear | |
| Other: | | Other: | |

| What Happened After the Seizure? | | | |
|---|---|---|---|
| Wobbly | | Weakness in the limbs | |
| Blindness | | Sniffing | |
| Pacing | | Disorientated | |
| Sleepy / tired | | Clingy | |
| Behaviour change: Aggressive / Fearful | | Staring into space / standing in corners | |
| Other: | | Other: | |

| Possible Triggers | | | |
|---|---|---|---|
| Time of day | | Seizures were 'due' (regular interval) | |
| Missed / late medication | | Medication change | |
| Missed sleep | | Missed meal | |
| Exercise | | Temperature (too hot / cold) | |
| Sensory (Loud sounds / flashing lights etc.) | | Specific food. Please note: | |
| Other medication, treatments or supplements. Please note: | | Stressful event. Please describe: | |
| Other: | | Other: | |

# *Seizure Log*

Date: _____     Time: _____     Duration: _____

Location: _____

Seizure Type: _____

If this was a cluster how many seizures? _____

Was your dog: Asleep ☐   Awake ☐   Waking from sleep ☐

What happened during the seizure?

_____

_____

_____

What was happening around the time the seizure occurred?

_____

_____

_____

Was there an Aura or warning?  Yes ☐   No ☐   Describe: _____

_____

_____

Rescue medication if given: _____

Taken to vet? Yes ☐   No ☐   Detail: _____

How long did your dog take to recover? _____

Notes:

_____

_____

_____

_____

_____

_____

# *Seizure Log*

| What Happened During the Seizure? | | | |
|---|---|---|---|
| The seizures started with the head | | The seizure started with the limbs | |
| The seizures started on the left / right | | My dog fell down | |
| Stiff body | | Floppy body | |
| Leg paddling | | Shaking | |
| Frothing / drooling | | Chewing movements | |
| Urination | | Defecation | |
| Weakness or twitching in one part of body | | Twitching on one side of face | |
| My dog could see | | My dog could hear | |
| Other: | | Other: | |

| What Happened After the Seizure? | | | |
|---|---|---|---|
| Wobbly | | Weakness in the limbs | |
| Blindness | | Sniffing | |
| Pacing | | Disorientated | |
| Sleepy / tired | | Clingy | |
| Behaviour change: Aggressive / Fearful | | Staring into space / standing in corners | |
| Other: | | Other: | |

| Possible Triggers | | | |
|---|---|---|---|
| Time of day | | Seizures were 'due' (regular interval) | |
| Missed / late medication | | Medication change | |
| Missed sleep | | Missed meal | |
| Exercise | | Temperature (too hot / cold) | |
| Sensory (Loud sounds / flashing lights etc.) | | Specific food. Please note: | |
| Other medication, treatments or supplements. Please note: | | Stressful event. Please describe: | |
| Other: | | Other: | |

# *Seizure Log*

Date: _____  Time: _____  Duration: _____

Location: _____

Seizure Type: _____

If this was a cluster how many seizures? _____

Was your dog: Asleep ☐  Awake ☐  Waking from sleep ☐

What happened during the seizure? _____

_____

_____

_____

What was happening around the time the seizure occurred?

_____

_____

_____

Was there an Aura or warning?  Yes ☐  No ☐  Describe: _____

_____

_____

Rescue medication if given: _____

Taken to vet? Yes ☐  No ☐  Detail: _____

How long did your dog take to recover? _____

Notes: _____

_____

_____

_____

_____

_____

# *Seizure Log*

| What Happened During the Seizure? | | | |
|---|---|---|---|
| The seizures started with the head | | The seizure started with the limbs | |
| The seizures started on the left / right | | My dog fell down | |
| Stiff body | | Floppy body | |
| Leg paddling | | Shaking | |
| Frothing / drooling | | Chewing movements | |
| Urination | | Defecation | |
| Weakness or twitching in one part of body | | Twitching on one side of face | |
| My dog could see | | My dog could hear | |
| Other: | | Other: | |

| What Happened After the Seizure? | | | |
|---|---|---|---|
| Wobbly | | Weakness in the limbs | |
| Blindness | | Sniffing | |
| Pacing | | Disorientated | |
| Sleepy / tired | | Clingy | |
| Behaviour change: Aggressive / Fearful | | Staring into space / standing in corners | |
| Other: | | Other: | |

| Possible Triggers | | | |
|---|---|---|---|
| Time of day | | Seizures were 'due' (regular interval) | |
| Missed / late medication | | Medication change | |
| Missed sleep | | Missed meal | |
| Exercise | | Temperature (too hot / cold) | |
| Sensory (Loud sounds / flashing lights etc.) | | Specific food. Please note: | |
| Other medication, treatments or supplements. Please note: | | Stressful event. Please describe: | |
| Other: | | Other: | |

# *Seizure Log*

Date: _____ Time: _____ Duration: _____

Location: _____

Seizure Type: _____

If this was a cluster how many seizures? _____

Was your dog: Asleep ☐ Awake ☐ Waking from sleep ☐

What happened during the seizure? _____

_____

_____

What was happening around the time the seizure occurred?

_____

_____

Was there an Aura or warning? Yes ☐ No ☐ Describe: _____

_____

Rescue medication if given: _____

Taken to vet? Yes ☐ No ☐ Detail: _____

How long did your dog take to recover? _____

Notes:

_____

_____

_____

_____

_____

_____

# *Seizure Log*

| What Happened During the Seizure? | | |
|---|---|---|
| The seizures started with the head | The seizure started with the limbs | |
| The seizures started on the left / right | My dog fell down | |
| Stiff body | Floppy body | |
| Leg paddling | Shaking | |
| Frothing / drooling | Chewing movements | |
| Urination | Defecation | |
| Weakness or twitching in one part of body | Twitching on one side of face | |
| My dog could see | My dog could hear | |
| Other: | Other: | |

| What Happened After the Seizure? | | |
|---|---|---|
| Wobbly | Weakness in the limbs | |
| Blindness | Sniffing | |
| Pacing | Disorientated | |
| Sleepy / tired | Clingy | |
| Behaviour change: Aggressive / Fearful | Staring into space / standing in corners | |
| Other: | Other: | |

| Possible Triggers | | |
|---|---|---|
| Time of day | Seizures were 'due' (regular interval) | |
| Missed / late medication | Medication change | |
| Missed sleep | Missed meal | |
| Exercise | Temperature (too hot / cold) | |
| Sensory (Loud sounds / flashing lights etc.) | Specific food. Please note: | |
| Other medication, treatments or supplements. Please note: | Stressful event. Please describe: | |
| Other: | Other: | |

141

# *Seizure Log*

Date: _____ Time: _____ Duration: _____

Location: _____

Seizure Type: _____

If this was a cluster how many seizures? _____

Was your dog: Asleep ☐ Awake ☐ Waking from sleep ☐

What happened during the seizure? _____

_____

_____

What was happening around the time the seizure occurred?

_____

_____

Was there an Aura or warning? Yes ☐ No ☐ Describe: _____

_____

_____

Rescue medication if given: _____

Taken to vet? Yes ☐ No ☐ Detail: _____

How long did your dog take to recover? _____

Notes: _____

_____

_____

_____

_____

_____

# *Seizure Log*

## What Happened During the Seizure?

| | | |
|---|---|---|
| The seizures started with the head | The seizure started with the limbs | |
| The seizures started on the left / right | My dog fell down | |
| Stiff body | Floppy body | |
| Leg paddling | Shaking | |
| Frothing / drooling | Chewing movements | |
| Urination | Defecation | |
| Weakness or twitching in one part of body | Twitching on one side of face | |
| My dog could see | My dog could hear | |
| Other: | Other: | |

## What Happened After the Seizure?

| | | |
|---|---|---|
| Wobbly | Weakness in the limbs | |
| Blindness | Sniffing | |
| Pacing | Disorientated | |
| Sleepy / tired | Clingy | |
| Behaviour change: Aggressive / Fearful | Staring into space / standing in corners | |
| Other: | Other: | |

## Possible Triggers

| | | |
|---|---|---|
| Time of day | Seizures were 'due' (regular interval) | |
| Missed / late medication | Medication change | |
| Missed sleep | Missed meal | |
| Exercise | Temperature (too hot / cold) | |
| Sensory (Loud sounds / flashing lights etc.) | Specific food. Please note: | |
| Other medication, treatments or supplements. Please note: | Stressful event. Please describe: | |
| Other: | Other: | |

# *Seizure Log*

Date: _____ Time: _____ Duration: _____

Location: _____

Seizure Type: _____

If this was a cluster how many seizures? _____

Was your dog: Asleep ☐ Awake ☐ Waking from sleep ☐

What happened during the seizure? _____

_____

_____

What was happening around the time the seizure occurred?

_____

_____

Was there an Aura or warning? Yes ☐ No ☐ Describe: _____

_____

_____

Rescue medication if given: _____

Taken to vet? Yes ☐ No ☐ Detail: _____

How long did your dog take to recover? _____

Notes: _____

_____

_____

_____

_____

_____

# *Seizure Log*

| What Happened During the Seizure? | | |
|---|---|---|
| The seizures started with the head | The seizure started with the limbs | |
| The seizures started on the left / right | My dog fell down | |
| Stiff body | Floppy body | |
| Leg paddling | Shaking | |
| Frothing / drooling | Chewing movements | |
| Urination | Defecation | |
| Weakness or twitching in one part of body | Twitching on one side of face | |
| My dog could see | My dog could hear | |
| Other: | Other: | |

| What Happened After the Seizure? | | |
|---|---|---|
| Wobbly | Weakness in the limbs | |
| Blindness | Sniffing | |
| Pacing | Disorientated | |
| Sleepy / tired | Clingy | |
| Behaviour change: Aggressive / Fearful | Staring into space / standing in corners | |
| Other: | Other: | |

| Possible Triggers | | |
|---|---|---|
| Time of day | Seizures were 'due' (regular interval) | |
| Missed / late medication | Medication change | |
| Missed sleep | Missed meal | |
| Exercise | Temperature (too hot / cold) | |
| Sensory (Loud sounds / flashing lights etc.) | Specific food. Please note: | |
| Other medication, treatments or supplements. Please note: | Stressful event. Please describe: | |
| Other: | Other: | |

145

# *Seizure Log*

Date: .................................... Time: .................................... Duration: ....................................

Location: ....................................................................................................................

Seizure Type: ..............................................................................................................

If this was a cluster how many seizures? ...........................................................

Was your dog: Asleep ☐  Awake ☐  Waking from sleep ☐

What happened during the seizure? ...................................................................

........................................................................................................................

........................................................................................................................

What was happening around the time the seizure occurred?

........................................................................................................................

........................................................................................................................

Was there an Aura or warning?  Yes ☐  No ☐  Describe: ....................................

........................................................................................................................

Rescue medication if given: ...............................................................................

Taken to vet? Yes ☐  No ☐  Detail: ...................................................................

How long did your dog take to recover? ............................................................

Notes: ...........................................................................................................

........................................................................................................................

........................................................................................................................

........................................................................................................................

........................................................................................................................

........................................................................................................................

# Seizure Log

| What Happened During the Seizure? | | |
|---|---|---|
| The seizures started with the head | The seizure started with the limbs | |
| The seizures started on the left / right | My dog fell down | |
| Stiff body | Floppy body | |
| Leg paddling | Shaking | |
| Frothing / drooling | Chewing movements | |
| Urination | Defecation | |
| Weakness or twitching in one part of body | Twitching on one side of face | |
| My dog could see | My dog could hear | |
| Other: | Other: | |

| What Happened After the Seizure? | | |
|---|---|---|
| Wobbly | Weakness in the limbs | |
| Blindness | Sniffing | |
| Pacing | Disorientated | |
| Sleepy / tired | Clingy | |
| Behaviour change: Aggressive / Fearful | Staring into space / standing in corners | |
| Other: | Other: | |

| Possible Triggers | | |
|---|---|---|
| Time of day | Seizures were 'due' (regular interval) | |
| Missed / late medication | Medication change | |
| Missed sleep | Missed meal | |
| Exercise | Temperature (too hot / cold) | |
| Sensory (Loud sounds / flashing lights etc.) | Specific food. Please note: | |
| Other medication, treatments or supplements. Please note: | Stressful event. Please describe: | |
| Other: | Other: | |

# *Seizure Log*

Date: _____ Time: _____ Duration: _____

Location: _____

Seizure Type: _____

If this was a cluster how many seizures? _____

Was your dog: Asleep ☐ Awake ☐ Waking from sleep ☐

What happened during the seizure? _____

_____

_____

_____

What was happening around the time the seizure occurred?

_____

_____

_____

Was there an Aura or warning? Yes ☐ No ☐ Describe: _____

_____

_____

Rescue medication if given: _____

Taken to vet? Yes ☐ No ☐ Detail: _____

How long did your dog take to recover? _____

Notes: _____

_____

_____

_____

_____

_____

# *Seizure Log*

| What Happened During the Seizure? | | | |
|---|---|---|---|
| The seizures started with the head | | The seizure started with the limbs | |
| The seizures started on the left / right | | My dog fell down | |
| Stiff body | | Floppy body | |
| Leg paddling | | Shaking | |
| Frothing / drooling | | Chewing movements | |
| Urination | | Defecation | |
| Weakness or twitching in one part of body | | Twitching on one side of face | |
| My dog could see | | My dog could hear | |
| Other: | | Other: | |

| What Happened After the Seizure? | | | |
|---|---|---|---|
| Wobbly | | Weakness in the limbs | |
| Blindness | | Sniffing | |
| Pacing | | Disorientated | |
| Sleepy / tired | | Clingy | |
| Behaviour change: Aggressive / Fearful | | Staring into space / standing in corners | |
| Other: | | Other: | |

| Possible Triggers | | | |
|---|---|---|---|
| Time of day | | Seizures were 'due' (regular interval) | |
| Missed / late medication | | Medication change | |
| Missed sleep | | Missed meal | |
| Exercise | | Temperature (too hot / cold) | |
| Sensory (Loud sounds / flashing lights etc.) | | Specific food. Please note: | |
| Other medication, treatments or supplements. Please note: | | Stressful event. Please describe: | |
| Other: | | Other: | |

# *Seizure Log*

Date: _____    Time: _____    Duration: _____

Location: ...................................................................................................

Seizure Type: ............................................................................................

If this was a cluster how many seizures? ...........................................

Was your dog: Asleep ☐   Awake ☐   Waking from sleep ☐

What happened during the seizure? ....................................................

.....................................................................................................................

.....................................................................................................................

.....................................................................................................................

What was happening around the time the seizure occurred?

.....................................................................................................................

.....................................................................................................................

.....................................................................................................................

Was there an Aura or warning?  Yes ☐  No ☐  Describe: ...................

.....................................................................................................................

.....................................................................................................................

Rescue medication if given: ..................................................................

Taken to vet? Yes ☐  No ☐  Detail: ...................................................

How long did your dog take to recover? ...........................................

Notes: .......................................................................................................

.....................................................................................................................

.....................................................................................................................

.....................................................................................................................

.....................................................................................................................

.....................................................................................................................

# *Seizure Log*

| What Happened During the Seizure? | | |
|---|---|---|
| The seizures started with the head | The seizure started with the limbs | |
| The seizures started on the left / right | My dog fell down | |
| Stiff body | Floppy body | |
| Leg paddling | Shaking | |
| Frothing / drooling | Chewing movements | |
| Urination | Defecation | |
| Weakness or twitching in one part of body | Twitching on one side of face | |
| My dog could see | My dog could hear | |
| Other: | Other: | |

| What Happened After the Seizure? | | |
|---|---|---|
| Wobbly | Weakness in the limbs | |
| Blindness | Sniffing | |
| Pacing | Disorientated | |
| Sleepy / tired | Clingy | |
| Behaviour change: Aggressive / Fearful | Staring into space / standing in corners | |
| Other: | Other: | |

| Possible Triggers | | |
|---|---|---|
| Time of day | Seizures were 'due' (regular interval) | |
| Missed / late medication | Medication change | |
| Missed sleep | Missed meal | |
| Exercise | Temperature (too hot / cold) | |
| Sensory (Loud sounds / flashing lights etc.) | Specific food. Please note: | |
| Other medication, treatments or supplements. Please note: | Stressful event. Please describe: | |
| Other: | Other: | |

151

# *Seizure Log*

Date: _____ Time: _____ Duration: _____

Location: _____

Seizure Type: _____

If this was a cluster how many seizures? _____

Was your dog: Asleep ☐ Awake ☐ Waking from sleep ☐

What happened during the seizure? _____

_____

_____

_____

What was happening around the time the seizure occurred?

_____

_____

_____

Was there an Aura or warning? Yes ☐ No ☐ Describe: _____

_____

_____

Rescue medication if given: _____

Taken to vet? Yes ☐ No ☐ Detail: _____

How long did your dog take to recover? _____

Notes: _____

_____

_____

_____

_____

_____

_____

# Seizure Log

| What Happened During the Seizure? | | |
|---|---|---|
| The seizures started with the head | The seizure started with the limbs | |
| The seizures started on the left / right | My dog fell down | |
| Stiff body | Floppy body | |
| Leg paddling | Shaking | |
| Frothing / drooling | Chewing movements | |
| Urination | Defecation | |
| Weakness or twitching in one part of body | Twitching on one side of face | |
| My dog could see | My dog could hear | |
| Other: | Other: | |

| What Happened After the Seizure? | | |
|---|---|---|
| Wobbly | Weakness in the limbs | |
| Blindness | Sniffing | |
| Pacing | Disorientated | |
| Sleepy / tired | Clingy | |
| Behaviour change: Aggressive / Fearful | Staring into space / standing in corners | |
| Other: | Other: | |

| Possible Triggers | | |
|---|---|---|
| Time of day | Seizures were 'due' (regular interval) | |
| Missed / late medication | Medication change | |
| Missed sleep | Missed meal | |
| Exercise | Temperature (too hot / cold) | |
| Sensory (Loud sounds / flashing lights etc.) | Specific food. Please note: | |
| Other medication, treatments or supplements. Please note: | Stressful event. Please describe: | |
| Other: | Other: | |

153

# *Seizure Log*

Date: _____    Time: _____    Duration: _____

Location: ...................................................................................................

Seizure Type: ............................................................................................

If this was a cluster how many seizures? ................................................

Was your dog: Asleep ☐   Awake ☐   Waking from sleep ☐

What happened during the seizure? ....................................................

..................................................................................................................

..................................................................................................................

..................................................................................................................

What was happening around the time the seizure occurred?

..................................................................................................................

..................................................................................................................

..................................................................................................................

Was there an Aura or warning?  Yes ☐   No ☐   Describe: ................

..................................................................................................................

..................................................................................................................

Rescue medication if given: ..............................................................

Taken to vet? Yes ☐   No ☐   Detail: ...............................................

How long did your dog take to recover? ............................................

Notes: .......................................................................................................

..................................................................................................................

..................................................................................................................

..................................................................................................................

..................................................................................................................

..................................................................................................................

# Seizure Log

| What Happened During the Seizure? | | | |
|---|---|---|---|
| The seizures started with the head | | The seizure started with the limbs | |
| The seizures started on the left / right | | My dog fell down | |
| Stiff body | | Floppy body | |
| Leg paddling | | Shaking | |
| Frothing / drooling | | Chewing movements | |
| Urination | | Defecation | |
| Weakness or twitching in one part of body | | Twitching on one side of face | |
| My dog could see | | My dog could hear | |
| Other: | | Other: | |

| What Happened After the Seizure? | | | |
|---|---|---|---|
| Wobbly | | Weakness in the limbs | |
| Blindness | | Sniffing | |
| Pacing | | Disorientated | |
| Sleepy / tired | | Clingy | |
| Behaviour change: Aggressive / Fearful | | Staring into space / standing in corners | |
| Other: | | Other: | |

| Possible Triggers | | | |
|---|---|---|---|
| Time of day | | Seizures were 'due' (regular interval) | |
| Missed / late medication | | Medication change | |
| Missed sleep | | Missed meal | |
| Exercise | | Temperature (too hot / cold) | |
| Sensory (Loud sounds / flashing lights etc.) | | Specific food. Please note: | |
| Other medication, treatments or supplements. Please note: | | Stressful event. Please describe: | |
| Other: | | Other: | |

# *Seizure Log*

Date: _____ Time: _____ Duration: _____

Location: _____

Seizure Type: _____

If this was a cluster how many seizures? _____

Was your dog: Asleep ☐ Awake ☐ Waking from sleep ☐

What happened during the seizure?

_____

_____

What was happening around the time the seizure occurred?

_____

_____

Was there an Aura or warning? Yes ☐ No ☐ Describe: _____

_____

Rescue medication if given: _____

Taken to vet? Yes ☐ No ☐ Detail: _____

How long did your dog take to recover? _____

Notes:

_____

_____

_____

_____

_____

# Seizure Log

| What Happened During the Seizure? | | |
|---|---|---|
| The seizures started with the head | The seizure started with the limbs | |
| The seizures started on the left / right | My dog fell down | |
| Stiff body | Floppy body | |
| Leg paddling | Shaking | |
| Frothing / drooling | Chewing movements | |
| Urination | Defecation | |
| Weakness or twitching in one part of body | Twitching on one side of face | |
| My dog could see | My dog could hear | |
| Other: | Other: | |

| What Happened After the Seizure? | | |
|---|---|---|
| Wobbly | Weakness in the limbs | |
| Blindness | Sniffing | |
| Pacing | Disorientated | |
| Sleepy / tired | Clingy | |
| Behaviour change: Aggressive / Fearful | Staring into space / standing in corners | |
| Other: | Other: | |

| Possible Triggers | | |
|---|---|---|
| Time of day | Seizures were 'due' (regular interval) | |
| Missed / late medication | Medication change | |
| Missed sleep | Missed meal | |
| Exercise | Temperature (too hot / cold) | |
| Sensory (Loud sounds / flashing lights etc.) | Specific food. Please note: | |
| Other medication, treatments or supplements. Please note: | Stressful event. Please describe: | |
| Other: | Other: | |

157

# *Seizure Log*

Date: _____ Time: _____ Duration: _____

Location: _____

Seizure Type: _____

If this was a cluster how many seizures? _____

Was your dog: Asleep ☐  Awake ☐  Waking from sleep ☐

What happened during the seizure? _____

_____

_____

_____

What was happening around the time the seizure occurred?

_____

_____

_____

Was there an Aura or warning?  Yes ☐  No ☐  Describe: _____

_____

_____

Rescue medication if given: _____

Taken to vet? Yes ☐  No ☐  Detail: _____

How long did your dog take to recover? _____

Notes: _____

_____

_____

_____

_____

_____

# Seizure Log

| What Happened During the Seizure? | | |
|---|---|---|
| The seizures started with the head | The seizure started with the limbs | |
| The seizures started on the left / right | My dog fell down | |
| Stiff body | Floppy body | |
| Leg paddling | Shaking | |
| Frothing / drooling | Chewing movements | |
| Urination | Defecation | |
| Weakness or twitching in one part of body | Twitching on one side of face | |
| My dog could see | My dog could hear | |
| Other: | Other: | |

| What Happened After the Seizure? | | |
|---|---|---|
| Wobbly | Weakness in the limbs | |
| Blindness | Sniffing | |
| Pacing | Disorientated | |
| Sleepy / tired | Clingy | |
| Behaviour change: Aggressive / Fearful | Staring into space / standing in corners | |
| Other: | Other: | |

| Possible Triggers | | |
|---|---|---|
| Time of day | Seizures were 'due' (regular interval) | |
| Missed / late medication | Medication change | |
| Missed sleep | Missed meal | |
| Exercise | Temperature (too hot / cold) | |
| Sensory (Loud sounds / flashing lights etc.) | Specific food. Please note: | |
| Other medication, treatments or supplements. Please note: | Stressful event. Please describe: | |
| Other: | Other: | |

159

# *Seizure Log*

Date: _____   Time: _____   Duration: _____

Location: _____

Seizure Type: _____

If this was a cluster how many seizures? _____

Was your dog: Asleep ☐   Awake ☐   Waking from sleep ☐

What happened during the seizure? _____

_____

_____

_____

What was happening around the time the seizure occurred?

_____

_____

Was there an Aura or warning?  Yes ☐   No ☐   Describe: _____

_____

_____

Rescue medication if given: _____

Taken to vet? Yes ☐   No ☐   Detail: _____

How long did your dog take to recover? _____

Notes: _____

_____

_____

_____

_____

_____

# Seizure Log

| What Happened During the Seizure? | | |
|---|---|---|
| The seizures started with the head | The seizure started with the limbs | |
| The seizures started on the left / right | My dog fell down | |
| Stiff body | Floppy body | |
| Leg paddling | Shaking | |
| Frothing / drooling | Chewing movements | |
| Urination | Defecation | |
| Weakness or twitching in one part of body | Twitching on one side of face | |
| My dog could see | My dog could hear | |
| Other: | Other: | |

| What Happened After the Seizure? | | |
|---|---|---|
| Wobbly | Weakness in the limbs | |
| Blindness | Sniffing | |
| Pacing | Disorientated | |
| Sleepy / tired | Clingy | |
| Behaviour change: Aggressive / Fearful | Staring into space / standing in corners | |
| Other: | Other: | |

| Possible Triggers | | |
|---|---|---|
| Time of day | Seizures were 'due' (regular interval) | |
| Missed / late medication | Medication change | |
| Missed sleep | Missed meal | |
| Exercise | Temperature (too hot / cold) | |
| Sensory (Loud sounds / flashing lights etc.) | Specific food. Please note: | |
| Other medication, treatments or supplements. Please note: | Stressful event. Please describe: | |
| Other: | Other: | |

161

# *Seizure Log*

Date: _____ Time: _____ Duration: _____

Location: _____

Seizure Type: _____

If this was a cluster how many seizures? _____

Was your dog: Asleep ☐ Awake ☐ Waking from sleep ☐

What happened during the seizure? _____

_____

_____

_____

What was happening around the time the seizure occurred?

_____

_____

_____

Was there an Aura or warning? Yes ☐ No ☐ Describe: _____

_____

_____

Rescue medication if given: _____

Taken to vet? Yes ☐ No ☐ Detail: _____

How long did your dog take to recover? _____

Notes: _____

_____

_____

_____

_____

_____

_____

# *Seizure Log*

| What Happened During the Seizure? | | | |
|---|---|---|---|
| The seizures started with the head | | The seizure started with the limbs | |
| The seizures started on the left / right | | My dog fell down | |
| Stiff body | | Floppy body | |
| Leg paddling | | Shaking | |
| Frothing / drooling | | Chewing movements | |
| Urination | | Defecation | |
| Weakness or twitching in one part of body | | Twitching on one side of face | |
| My dog could see | | My dog could hear | |
| Other: | | Other: | |

| What Happened After the Seizure? | | | |
|---|---|---|---|
| Wobbly | | Weakness in the limbs | |
| Blindness | | Sniffing | |
| Pacing | | Disorientated | |
| Sleepy / tired | | Clingy | |
| Behaviour change: Aggressive / Fearful | | Staring into space / standing in corners | |
| Other: | | Other: | |

| Possible Triggers | | | |
|---|---|---|---|
| Time of day | | Seizures were 'due' (regular interval) | |
| Missed / late medication | | Medication change | |
| Missed sleep | | Missed meal | |
| Exercise | | Temperature (too hot / cold) | |
| Sensory (Loud sounds / flashing lights etc.) | | Specific food. Please note: | |
| Other medication, treatments or supplements. Please note: | | Stressful event. Please describe: | |
| Other: | | Other: | |

163

# Seizure Log

Date: _____    Time: _____    Duration: _____

Location: _____

Seizure Type: _____

If this was a cluster how many seizures? _____

Was your dog: Asleep ☐  Awake ☐  Waking from sleep ☐

What happened during the seizure? _____

_____

_____

What was happening around the time the seizure occurred?

_____

_____

Was there an Aura or warning?  Yes ☐  No ☐  Describe: _____

_____

Rescue medication if given: _____

Taken to vet? Yes ☐  No ☐  Detail: _____

How long did your dog take to recover? _____

Notes: _____

_____

_____

_____

_____

_____

# *Seizure Log*

| What Happened During the Seizure? | | | |
|---|---|---|---|
| The seizures started with the head | | The seizure started with the limbs | |
| The seizures started on the left / right | | My dog fell down | |
| Stiff body | | Floppy body | |
| Leg paddling | | Shaking | |
| Frothing / drooling | | Chewing movements | |
| Urination | | Defecation | |
| Weakness or twitching in one part of body | | Twitching on one side of face | |
| My dog could see | | My dog could hear | |
| Other: | | Other: | |

| What Happened After the Seizure? | | | |
|---|---|---|---|
| Wobbly | | Weakness in the limbs | |
| Blindness | | Sniffing | |
| Pacing | | Disorientated | |
| Sleepy / tired | | Clingy | |
| Behaviour change: Aggressive / Fearful | | Staring into space / standing in corners | |
| Other: | | Other: | |

| Possible Triggers | | | |
|---|---|---|---|
| Time of day | | Seizures were 'due' (regular interval) | |
| Missed / late medication | | Medication change | |
| Missed sleep | | Missed meal | |
| Exercise | | Temperature (too hot / cold) | |
| Sensory (Loud sounds / flashing lights etc.) | | Specific food. Please note: | |
| Other medication, treatments or supplements. Please note: | | Stressful event. Please describe: | |
| Other: | | Other: | |

# *Seizure Log*

Date: _____ Time: _____ Duration: _____

Location: _____

Seizure Type: _____

If this was a cluster how many seizures? _____

Was your dog: Asleep ☐  Awake ☐  Waking from sleep ☐

What happened during the seizure? _____

_____

_____

What was happening around the time the seizure occurred?

_____

_____

Was there an Aura or warning?  Yes ☐  No ☐  Describe: _____

_____

Rescue medication if given: _____

Taken to vet? Yes ☐  No ☐  Detail: _____

How long did your dog take to recover? _____

Notes: _____

_____

_____

_____

_____

_____

# *Seizure Log*

| What Happened During the Seizure? | | | |
|---|---|---|---|
| The seizures started with the head | | The seizure started with the limbs | |
| The seizures started on the left / right | | My dog fell down | |
| Stiff body | | Floppy body | |
| Leg paddling | | Shaking | |
| Frothing / drooling | | Chewing movements | |
| Urination | | Defecation | |
| Weakness or twitching in one part of body | | Twitching on one side of face | |
| My dog could see | | My dog could hear | |
| Other: | | Other: | |

| What Happened After the Seizure? | | | |
|---|---|---|---|
| Wobbly | | Weakness in the limbs | |
| Blindness | | Sniffing | |
| Pacing | | Disorientated | |
| Sleepy / tired | | Clingy | |
| Behaviour change: Aggressive / Fearful | | Staring into space / standing in corners | |
| Other: | | Other: | |

| Possible Triggers | | | |
|---|---|---|---|
| Time of day | | Seizures were 'due' (regular interval) | |
| Missed / late medication | | Medication change | |
| Missed sleep | | Missed meal | |
| Exercise | | Temperature (too hot / cold) | |
| Sensory (Loud sounds / flashing lights etc.) | | Specific food. Please note: | |
| Other medication, treatments or supplements. Please note: | | Stressful event. Please describe: | |
| Other: | | Other: | |

# *Seizure Log*

Date: _____  Time: _____  Duration: _____

Location: _____

Seizure Type: _____

If this was a cluster how many seizures? _____

Was your dog: Asleep ☐  Awake ☐  Waking from sleep ☐

What happened during the seizure? _____

_____

_____

_____

What was happening around the time the seizure occurred?

_____

_____

_____

Was there an Aura or warning?  Yes ☐  No ☐  Describe: _____

_____

_____

Rescue medication if given: _____

Taken to vet? Yes ☐  No ☐  Detail: _____

How long did your dog take to recover? _____

Notes: _____

_____

_____

_____

_____

_____

_____

# Seizure Log

| What Happened During the Seizure? | | | |
|---|---|---|---|
| The seizures started with the head | | The seizure started with the limbs | |
| The seizures started on the left / right | | My dog fell down | |
| Stiff body | | Floppy body | |
| Leg paddling | | Shaking | |
| Frothing / drooling | | Chewing movements | |
| Urination | | Defecation | |
| Weakness or twitching in one part of body | | Twitching on one side of face | |
| My dog could see | | My dog could hear | |
| Other: | | Other: | |

| What Happened After the Seizure? | | | |
|---|---|---|---|
| Wobbly | | Weakness in the limbs | |
| Blindness | | Sniffing | |
| Pacing | | Disorientated | |
| Sleepy / tired | | Clingy | |
| Behaviour change: Aggressive / Fearful | | Staring into space / standing in corners | |
| Other: | | Other: | |

| Possible Triggers | | | |
|---|---|---|---|
| Time of day | | Seizures were 'due' (regular interval) | |
| Missed / late medication | | Medication change | |
| Missed sleep | | Missed meal | |
| Exercise | | Temperature (too hot / cold) | |
| Sensory (Loud sounds / flashing lights etc.) | | Specific food. Please note: | |
| Other medication, treatments or supplements. Please note: | | Stressful event. Please describe: | |
| Other: | | Other: | |

# *Seizure Log*

Date: _____ Time: _____ Duration: _____

Location: _____

Seizure Type: _____

If this was a cluster how many seizures? _____

Was your dog: Asleep ☐ Awake ☐ Waking from sleep ☐

What happened during the seizure? _____

_____

_____

What was happening around the time the seizure occurred?

_____

_____

Was there an Aura or warning? Yes ☐ No ☐ Describe: _____

_____

Rescue medication if given: _____

Taken to vet? Yes ☐ No ☐ Detail: _____

How long did your dog take to recover? _____

Notes: _____

_____

_____

_____

_____

# Seizure Log

| What Happened During the Seizure? | | | |
|---|---|---|---|
| The seizures started with the head | | The seizure started with the limbs | |
| The seizures started on the left / right | | My dog fell down | |
| Stiff body | | Floppy body | |
| Leg paddling | | Shaking | |
| Frothing / drooling | | Chewing movements | |
| Urination | | Defecation | |
| Weakness or twitching in one part of body | | Twitching on one side of face | |
| My dog could see | | My dog could hear | |
| Other: | | Other: | |

| What Happened After the Seizure? | | | |
|---|---|---|---|
| Wobbly | | Weakness in the limbs | |
| Blindness | | Sniffing | |
| Pacing | | Disorientated | |
| Sleepy / tired | | Clingy | |
| Behaviour change: Aggressive / Fearful | | Staring into space / standing in corners | |
| Other: | | Other: | |

| Possible Triggers | | | |
|---|---|---|---|
| Time of day | | Seizures were 'due' (regular interval) | |
| Missed / late medication | | Medication change | |
| Missed sleep | | Missed meal | |
| Exercise | | Temperature (too hot / cold) | |
| Sensory (Loud sounds / flashing lights etc.) | | Specific food. Please note: | |
| Other medication, treatments or supplements. Please note: | | Stressful event. Please describe: | |
| Other: | | Other: | |

# *Seizure Log*

Date: _____    Time: _____    Duration: _____

Location: _____

Seizure Type: _____

If this was a cluster how many seizures? _____

Was your dog: Asleep ☐   Awake ☐   Waking from sleep ☐

What happened during the seizure? _____

_____

_____

What was happening around the time the seizure occurred?

_____

_____

Was there an Aura or warning?  Yes ☐   No ☐   Describe: _____

_____

_____

Rescue medication if given: _____

Taken to vet? Yes ☐   No ☐   Detail: _____

How long did your dog take to recover? _____

Notes: _____

_____

_____

_____

_____

_____

# Seizure Log

| What Happened During the Seizure? | | | |
|---|---|---|---|
| The seizures started with the head | | The seizure started with the limbs | |
| The seizures started on the left / right | | My dog fell down | |
| Stiff body | | Floppy body | |
| Leg paddling | | Shaking | |
| Frothing / drooling | | Chewing movements | |
| Urination | | Defecation | |
| Weakness or twitching in one part of body | | Twitching on one side of face | |
| My dog could see | | My dog could hear | |
| Other: | | Other: | |

| What Happened After the Seizure? | | | |
|---|---|---|---|
| Wobbly | | Weakness in the limbs | |
| Blindness | | Sniffing | |
| Pacing | | Disorientated | |
| Sleepy / tired | | Clingy | |
| Behaviour change: Aggressive / Fearful | | Staring into space / standing in corners | |
| Other: | | Other: | |

| Possible Triggers | | | |
|---|---|---|---|
| Time of day | | Seizures were 'due' (regular interval) | |
| Missed / late medication | | Medication change | |
| Missed sleep | | Missed meal | |
| Exercise | | Temperature (too hot / cold) | |
| Sensory (Loud sounds / flashing lights etc.) | | Specific food. Please note: | |
| Other medication, treatments or supplements. Please note: | | Stressful event. Please describe: | |
| Other: | | Other: | |

173

# *Seizure Log*

Date: _____  Time: _____  Duration: _____

Location: _____

Seizure Type: _____

If this was a cluster how many seizures? _____

Was your dog: Asleep ☐  Awake ☐  Waking from sleep ☐

What happened during the seizure?

_____

_____

_____

What was happening around the time the seizure occurred?

_____

_____

_____

Was there an Aura or warning?  Yes ☐  No ☐  Describe: _____

_____

_____

Rescue medication if given: _____

Taken to vet? Yes ☐  No ☐  Detail: _____

How long did your dog take to recover? _____

Notes:

_____

_____

_____

_____

_____

_____

# Seizure Log

| What Happened During the Seizure? | | | |
|---|---|---|---|
| The seizures started with the head | | The seizure started with the limbs | |
| The seizures started on the left / right | | My dog fell down | |
| Stiff body | | Floppy body | |
| Leg paddling | | Shaking | |
| Frothing / drooling | | Chewing movements | |
| Urination | | Defecation | |
| Weakness or twitching in one part of body | | Twitching on one side of face | |
| My dog could see | | My dog could hear | |
| Other: | | Other: | |

| What Happened After the Seizure? | | | |
|---|---|---|---|
| Wobbly | | Weakness in the limbs | |
| Blindness | | Sniffing | |
| Pacing | | Disorientated | |
| Sleepy / tired | | Clingy | |
| Behaviour change: Aggressive / Fearful | | Staring into space / standing in corners | |
| Other: | | Other: | |

| Possible Triggers | | | |
|---|---|---|---|
| Time of day | | Seizures were 'due' (regular interval) | |
| Missed / late medication | | Medication change | |
| Missed sleep | | Missed meal | |
| Exercise | | Temperature (too hot / cold) | |
| Sensory (Loud sounds / flashing lights etc.) | | Specific food. Please note: | |
| Other medication, treatments or supplements. Please note: | | Stressful event. Please describe: | |
| Other: | | Other: | |

175

# *Seizure Log*

Date: _____     Time: _____     Duration: _____

Location: _____

Seizure Type: _____

If this was a cluster how many seizures? _____

Was your dog: Asleep ☐   Awake ☐   Waking from sleep ☐

What happened during the seizure?

_____

_____

_____

What was happening around the time the seizure occurred?

_____

_____

_____

Was there an Aura or warning?   Yes ☐   No ☐   Describe: _____

_____

_____

Rescue medication if given: _____

Taken to vet? Yes ☐   No ☐   Detail: _____

How long did your dog take to recover? _____

Notes:

_____

_____

_____

_____

_____

# *Seizure Log*

| What Happened During the Seizure? | | | |
|---|---|---|---|
| The seizures started with the head | | The seizure started with the limbs | |
| The seizures started on the left / right | | My dog fell down | |
| Stiff body | | Floppy body | |
| Leg paddling | | Shaking | |
| Frothing / drooling | | Chewing movements | |
| Urination | | Defecation | |
| Weakness or twitching in one part of body | | Twitching on one side of face | |
| My dog could see | | My dog could hear | |
| Other: | | Other: | |

| What Happened After the Seizure? | | | |
|---|---|---|---|
| Wobbly | | Weakness in the limbs | |
| Blindness | | Sniffing | |
| Pacing | | Disorientated | |
| Sleepy / tired | | Clingy | |
| Behaviour change: Aggressive / Fearful | | Staring into space / standing in corners | |
| Other: | | Other: | |

| Possible Triggers | | | |
|---|---|---|---|
| Time of day | | Seizures were 'due' (regular interval) | |
| Missed / late medication | | Medication change | |
| Missed sleep | | Missed meal | |
| Exercise | | Temperature (too hot / cold) | |
| Sensory (Loud sounds / flashing lights etc.) | | Specific food. Please note: | |
| Other medication, treatments or supplements. Please note: | | Stressful event. Please describe: | |
| Other: | | Other: | |

# *Seizure Log*

Date: _____  Time: _____  Duration: _____

Location: _____

Seizure Type: _____

If this was a cluster how many seizures? _____

Was your dog: Asleep ☐  Awake ☐  Waking from sleep ☐

What happened during the seizure? _____

_____

_____

What was happening around the time the seizure occurred?

_____

_____

Was there an Aura or warning?  Yes ☐  No ☐  Describe: _____

_____

Rescue medication if given: _____

Taken to vet? Yes ☐  No ☐  Detail: _____

How long did your dog take to recover? _____

Notes: _____

_____

_____

_____

_____

# *Seizure Log*

| What Happened During the Seizure? | | | |
|---|:---:|---|:---:|
| The seizures started with the head | | The seizure started with the limbs | |
| The seizures started on the left / right | | My dog fell down | |
| Stiff body | | Floppy body | |
| Leg paddling | | Shaking | |
| Frothing / drooling | | Chewing movements | |
| Urination | | Defecation | |
| Weakness or twitching in one part of body | | Twitching on one side of face | |
| My dog could see | | My dog could hear | |
| Other: | | Other: | |

| What Happened After the Seizure? | | | |
|---|:---:|---|:---:|
| Wobbly | | Weakness in the limbs | |
| Blindness | | Sniffing | |
| Pacing | | Disorientated | |
| Sleepy / tired | | Clingy | |
| Behaviour change: Aggressive / Fearful | | Staring into space / standing in corners | |
| Other: | | Other: | |

| Possible Triggers | | | |
|---|:---:|---|:---:|
| Time of day | | Seizures were 'due' (regular interval) | |
| Missed / late medication | | Medication change | |
| Missed sleep | | Missed meal | |
| Exercise | | Temperature (too hot / cold) | |
| Sensory (Loud sounds / flashing lights etc.) | | Specific food. Please note: | |
| Other medication, treatments or supplements. Please note: | | Stressful event. Please describe: | |
| Other: | | Other: | |

# *Seizure Log*

Date: _____     Time: _____     Duration: _____

Location: _____

Seizure Type: _____

If this was a cluster how many seizures? _____

Was your dog: Asleep ☐   Awake ☐   Waking from sleep ☐

What happened during the seizure?

_____

_____

What was happening around the time the seizure occurred?

_____

_____

Was there an Aura or warning?  Yes ☐  No ☐  Describe: _____

_____

Rescue medication if given: _____

Taken to vet? Yes ☐  No ☐  Detail: _____

How long did your dog take to recover? _____

Notes:

_____

_____

_____

_____

_____

# Seizure Log

| What Happened During the Seizure? | | |
|---|---|---|
| The seizures started with the head | The seizure started with the limbs | |
| The seizures started on the left / right | My dog fell down | |
| Stiff body | Floppy body | |
| Leg paddling | Shaking | |
| Frothing / drooling | Chewing movements | |
| Urination | Defecation | |
| Weakness or twitching in one part of body | Twitching on one side of face | |
| My dog could see | My dog could hear | |
| Other: | Other: | |

| What Happened After the Seizure? | | |
|---|---|---|
| Wobbly | Weakness in the limbs | |
| Blindness | Sniffing | |
| Pacing | Disorientated | |
| Sleepy / tired | Clingy | |
| Behaviour change: Aggressive / Fearful | Staring into space / standing in corners | |
| Other: | Other: | |

| Possible Triggers | | |
|---|---|---|
| Time of day | Seizures were 'due' (regular interval) | |
| Missed / late medication | Medication change | |
| Missed sleep | Missed meal | |
| Exercise | Temperature (too hot / cold) | |
| Sensory (Loud sounds / flashing lights etc.) | Specific food. Please note: | |
| Other medication, treatments or supplements. Please note: | Stressful event. Please describe: | |
| Other: | Other: | |

# *Seizure Log*

Date: _____ Time: _____ Duration: _____

Location: _____

Seizure Type: _____

If this was a cluster how many seizures? _____

Was your dog: Asleep ☐  Awake ☐  Waking from sleep ☐

What happened during the seizure?

_____

_____

_____

What was happening around the time the seizure occurred?

_____

_____

Was there an Aura or warning?  Yes ☐  No ☐  Describe: _____

_____

Rescue medication if given: _____

Taken to vet? Yes ☐  No ☐  Detail: _____

How long did your dog take to recover? _____

Notes:

_____

_____

_____

_____

_____

# Seizure Log

| What Happened During the Seizure? | | | |
|---|---|---|---|
| The seizures started with the head | | The seizure started with the limbs | |
| The seizures started on the left / right | | My dog fell down | |
| Stiff body | | Floppy body | |
| Leg paddling | | Shaking | |
| Frothing / drooling | | Chewing movements | |
| Urination | | Defecation | |
| Weakness or twitching in one part of body | | Twitching on one side of face | |
| My dog could see | | My dog could hear | |
| Other: | | Other: | |

| What Happened After the Seizure? | | | |
|---|---|---|---|
| Wobbly | | Weakness in the limbs | |
| Blindness | | Sniffing | |
| Pacing | | Disorientated | |
| Sleepy / tired | | Clingy | |
| Behaviour change: Aggressive / Fearful | | Staring into space / standing in corners | |
| Other: | | Other: | |

| Possible Triggers | | | |
|---|---|---|---|
| Time of day | | Seizures were 'due' (regular interval) | |
| Missed / late medication | | Medication change | |
| Missed sleep | | Missed meal | |
| Exercise | | Temperature (too hot / cold) | |
| Sensory (Loud sounds / flashing lights etc.) | | Specific food. Please note: | |
| Other medication, treatments or supplements. Please note: | | Stressful event. Please describe: | |
| Other: | | Other: | |

183

# *Seizure Log*

Date: _____    Time: _____    Duration: _____

Location: _____

Seizure Type: _____

If this was a cluster how many seizures? _____

Was your dog: Asleep ☐   Awake ☐   Waking from sleep ☐

What happened during the seizure? _____

_____

_____

What was happening around the time the seizure occurred?

_____

_____

Was there an Aura or warning?  Yes ☐   No ☐   Describe: _____

_____

Rescue medication if given: _____

Taken to vet? Yes ☐   No ☐   Detail: _____

How long did your dog take to recover? _____

Notes: _____

_____

_____

_____

_____

# *Seizure Log*

| What Happened During the Seizure? | | | |
|---|---|---|---|
| The seizures started with the head | | The seizure started with the limbs | |
| The seizures started on the left / right | | My dog fell down | |
| Stiff body | | Floppy body | |
| Leg paddling | | Shaking | |
| Frothing / drooling | | Chewing movements | |
| Urination | | Defecation | |
| Weakness or twitching in one part of body | | Twitching on one side of face | |
| My dog could see | | My dog could hear | |
| Other: | | Other: | |

| What Happened After the Seizure? | | | |
|---|---|---|---|
| Wobbly | | Weakness in the limbs | |
| Blindness | | Sniffing | |
| Pacing | | Disorientated | |
| Sleepy / tired | | Clingy | |
| Behaviour change: Aggressive / Fearful | | Staring into space / standing in corners | |
| Other: | | Other: | |

| Possible Triggers | | | |
|---|---|---|---|
| Time of day | | Seizures were 'due' (regular interval) | |
| Missed / late medication | | Medication change | |
| Missed sleep | | Missed meal | |
| Exercise | | Temperature (too hot / cold) | |
| Sensory (Loud sounds / flashing lights etc.) | | Specific food. Please note: | |
| Other medication, treatments or supplements. Please note: | | Stressful event. Please describe: | |
| Other: | | Other: | |

# *Seizure Log*

Date: _____  Time: _____  Duration: _____

Location: _____

Seizure Type: _____

If this was a cluster how many seizures? _____

Was your dog: Asleep ☐  Awake ☐  Waking from sleep ☐

What happened during the seizure? _____

_____

_____

_____

What was happening around the time the seizure occurred?

_____

_____

_____

Was there an Aura or warning?  Yes ☐  No ☐  Describe: _____

_____

_____

Rescue medication if given: _____

Taken to vet? Yes ☐  No ☐  Detail: _____

How long did your dog take to recover? _____

Notes: _____

_____

_____

_____

_____

_____

# *Seizure Log*

| What Happened During the Seizure? | | |
|---|---|---|
| The seizures started with the head | The seizure started with the limbs | |
| The seizures started on the left / right | My dog fell down | |
| Stiff body | Floppy body | |
| Leg paddling | Shaking | |
| Frothing / drooling | Chewing movements | |
| Urination | Defecation | |
| Weakness or twitching in one part of body | Twitching on one side of face | |
| My dog could see | My dog could hear | |
| Other: | Other: | |

| What Happened After the Seizure? | | |
|---|---|---|
| Wobbly | Weakness in the limbs | |
| Blindness | Sniffing | |
| Pacing | Disorientated | |
| Sleepy / tired | Clingy | |
| Behaviour change: Aggressive / Fearful | Staring into space / standing in corners | |
| Other: | Other: | |

| Possible Triggers | | |
|---|---|---|
| Time of day | Seizures were 'due' (regular interval) | |
| Missed / late medication | Medication change | |
| Missed sleep | Missed meal | |
| Exercise | Temperature (too hot / cold) | |
| Sensory (Loud sounds / flashing lights etc.) | Specific food. Please note: | |
| Other medication, treatments or supplements. Please note: | Stressful event. Please describe: | |
| Other: | Other: | |

187

# *Seizure Log*

Date: _____ Time: _____ Duration: _____

Location: _____

Seizure Type: _____

If this was a cluster how many seizures? _____

Was your dog: Asleep ☐ Awake ☐ Waking from sleep ☐

What happened during the seizure? _____

_____

_____

What was happening around the time the seizure occurred? _____

_____

_____

Was there an Aura or warning? Yes ☐ No ☐ Describe: _____

_____

_____

Rescue medication if given: _____

Taken to vet? Yes ☐ No ☐ Detail: _____

How long did your dog take to recover? _____

Notes: _____

_____

_____

_____

_____

_____

# Seizure Log

| What Happened During the Seizure? | | | |
|---|---|---|---|
| The seizures started with the head | | The seizure started with the limbs | |
| The seizures started on the left / right | | My dog fell down | |
| Stiff body | | Floppy body | |
| Leg paddling | | Shaking | |
| Frothing / drooling | | Chewing movements | |
| Urination | | Defecation | |
| Weakness or twitching in one part of body | | Twitching on one side of face | |
| My dog could see | | My dog could hear | |
| Other: | | Other: | |

| What Happened After the Seizure? | | | |
|---|---|---|---|
| Wobbly | | Weakness in the limbs | |
| Blindness | | Sniffing | |
| Pacing | | Disorientated | |
| Sleepy / tired | | Clingy | |
| Behaviour change: Aggressive / Fearful | | Staring into space / standing in corners | |
| Other: | | Other: | |

| Possible Triggers | | | |
|---|---|---|---|
| Time of day | | Seizures were 'due' (regular interval) | |
| Missed / late medication | | Medication change | |
| Missed sleep | | Missed meal | |
| Exercise | | Temperature (too hot / cold) | |
| Sensory (Loud sounds / flashing lights etc.) | | Specific food. Please note: | |
| Other medication, treatments or supplements. Please note: | | Stressful event. Please describe: | |
| Other: | | Other: | |

# *Seizure Log*

Date: _____  Time: _____  Duration: _____

Location: _____

Seizure Type: _____

If this was a cluster how many seizures? _____

Was your dog: Asleep ☐  Awake ☐  Waking from sleep ☐

What happened during the seizure? _____

_____

_____

_____

What was happening around the time the seizure occurred?

_____

_____

_____

Was there an Aura or warning? Yes ☐  No ☐  Describe: _____

_____

_____

Rescue medication if given: _____

Taken to vet? Yes ☐  No ☐  Detail: _____

How long did your dog take to recover? _____

Notes: _____

_____

_____

_____

_____

_____

# Seizure Log

| What Happened During the Seizure? | | | |
|---|---|---|---|
| The seizures started with the head | | The seizure started with the limbs | |
| The seizures started on the left / right | | My dog fell down | |
| Stiff body | | Floppy body | |
| Leg paddling | | Shaking | |
| Frothing / drooling | | Chewing movements | |
| Urination | | Defecation | |
| Weakness or twitching in one part of body | | Twitching on one side of face | |
| My dog could see | | My dog could hear | |
| Other: | | Other: | |

| What Happened After the Seizure? | | | |
|---|---|---|---|
| Wobbly | | Weakness in the limbs | |
| Blindness | | Sniffing | |
| Pacing | | Disorientated | |
| Sleepy / tired | | Clingy | |
| Behaviour change: Aggressive / Fearful | | Staring into space / standing in corners | |
| Other: | | Other: | |

| Possible Triggers | | | |
|---|---|---|---|
| Time of day | | Seizures were 'due' (regular interval) | |
| Missed / late medication | | Medication change | |
| Missed sleep | | Missed meal | |
| Exercise | | Temperature (too hot / cold) | |
| Sensory (Loud sounds / flashing lights etc.) | | Specific food. Please note: | |
| Other medication, treatments or supplements. Please note: | | Stressful event. Please describe: | |
| Other: | | Other: | |

# *Seizure Log*

Date: _____    Time: _____    Duration: _____

Location: _____

Seizure Type: _____

If this was a cluster how many seizures? _____

Was your dog: Asleep ☐   Awake ☐   Waking from sleep ☐

What happened during the seizure? _____

_____

_____

_____

What was happening around the time the seizure occurred?

_____

_____

_____

Was there an Aura or warning? Yes ☐  No ☐  Describe: _____

_____

_____

Rescue medication if given: _____

Taken to vet? Yes ☐  No ☐  Detail: _____

How long did your dog take to recover? _____

Notes: _____

_____

_____

_____

_____

_____

# Seizure Log

| What Happened During the Seizure? | | | |
|---|---|---|---|
| The seizures started with the head | | The seizure started with the limbs | |
| The seizures started on the left / right | | My dog fell down | |
| Stiff body | | Floppy body | |
| Leg paddling | | Shaking | |
| Frothing / drooling | | Chewing movements | |
| Urination | | Defecation | |
| Weakness or twitching in one part of body | | Twitching on one side of face | |
| My dog could see | | My dog could hear | |
| Other: | | Other: | |

| What Happened After the Seizure? | | | |
|---|---|---|---|
| Wobbly | | Weakness in the limbs | |
| Blindness | | Sniffing | |
| Pacing | | Disorientated | |
| Sleepy / tired | | Clingy | |
| Behaviour change: Aggressive / Fearful | | Staring into space / standing in corners | |
| Other: | | Other: | |

| Possible Triggers | | | |
|---|---|---|---|
| Time of day | | Seizures were 'due' (regular interval) | |
| Missed / late medication | | Medication change | |
| Missed sleep | | Missed meal | |
| Exercise | | Temperature (too hot / cold) | |
| Sensory (Loud sounds / flashing lights etc.) | | Specific food. Please note: | |
| Other medication, treatments or supplements. Please note: | | Stressful event. Please describe: | |
| Other: | | Other: | |

# *Seizure Log*

Date: _____ Time: _____ Duration: _____

Location: _____

Seizure Type: _____

If this was a cluster how many seizures? _____

Was your dog: Asleep ☐  Awake ☐  Waking from sleep ☐

What happened during the seizure? _____

_____

_____

_____

What was happening around the time the seizure occurred?

_____

_____

Was there an Aura or warning?  Yes ☐  No ☐  Describe: _____

_____

Rescue medication if given: _____

Taken to vet? Yes ☐  No ☐  Detail: _____

How long did your dog take to recover? _____

Notes: _____

_____

_____

_____

_____

_____

# *Seizure Log*

| What Happened During the Seizure? | | | |
|---|---|---|---|
| The seizures started with the head | | The seizure started with the limbs | |
| The seizures started on the left / right | | My dog fell down | |
| Stiff body | | Floppy body | |
| Leg paddling | | Shaking | |
| Frothing / drooling | | Chewing movements | |
| Urination | | Defecation | |
| Weakness or twitching in one part of body | | Twitching on one side of face | |
| My dog could see | | My dog could hear | |
| Other: | | Other: | |

| What Happened After the Seizure? | | | |
|---|---|---|---|
| Wobbly | | Weakness in the limbs | |
| Blindness | | Sniffing | |
| Pacing | | Disorientated | |
| Sleepy / tired | | Clingy | |
| Behaviour change: Aggressive / Fearful | | Staring into space / standing in corners | |
| Other: | | Other: | |

| Possible Triggers | | | |
|---|---|---|---|
| Time of day | | Seizures were 'due' (regular interval) | |
| Missed / late medication | | Medication change | |
| Missed sleep | | Missed meal | |
| Exercise | | Temperature (too hot / cold) | |
| Sensory (Loud sounds / flashing lights etc.) | | Specific food. Please note: | |
| Other medication, treatments or supplements. Please note: | | Stressful event. Please describe: | |
| Other: | | Other: | |

195

# *Seizure Log*

Date: _____  Time: _____  Duration: _____

Location: _____

Seizure Type: _____

If this was a cluster how many seizures? _____

Was your dog: Asleep ☐  Awake ☐  Waking from sleep ☐

What happened during the seizure? _____

_____

_____

_____

What was happening around the time the seizure occurred?

_____

_____

_____

Was there an Aura or warning?  Yes ☐  No ☐  Describe: _____

_____

_____

Rescue medication if given: _____

Taken to vet? Yes ☐  No ☐  Detail: _____

How long did your dog take to recover? _____

Notes: _____

_____

_____

_____

_____

_____

# Seizure Log

| What Happened During the Seizure? | | | |
|---|---|---|---|
| The seizures started with the head | | The seizure started with the limbs | |
| The seizures started on the left / right | | My dog fell down | |
| Stiff body | | Floppy body | |
| Leg paddling | | Shaking | |
| Frothing / drooling | | Chewing movements | |
| Urination | | Defecation | |
| Weakness or twitching in one part of body | | Twitching on one side of face | |
| My dog could see | | My dog could hear | |
| Other: | | Other: | |

| What Happened After the Seizure? | | | |
|---|---|---|---|
| Wobbly | | Weakness in the limbs | |
| Blindness | | Sniffing | |
| Pacing | | Disorientated | |
| Sleepy / tired | | Clingy | |
| Behaviour change: Aggressive / Fearful | | Staring into space / standing in corners | |
| Other: | | Other: | |

| Possible Triggers | | | |
|---|---|---|---|
| Time of day | | Seizures were 'due' (regular interval) | |
| Missed / late medication | | Medication change | |
| Missed sleep | | Missed meal | |
| Exercise | | Temperature (too hot / cold) | |
| Sensory (Loud sounds / flashing lights etc.) | | Specific food. Please note: | |
| Other medication, treatments or supplements. Please note: | | Stressful event. Please describe: | |
| Other: | | Other: | |

197

# *Seizure Log*

Date: _____     Time: _____     Duration: _____

Location: _____

Seizure Type: _____

If this was a cluster how many seizures? _____

Was your dog: Asleep ☐  Awake ☐  Waking from sleep ☐

What happened during the seizure? _____

_____

_____

What was happening around the time the seizure occurred? _____

_____

_____

Was there an Aura or warning? Yes ☐  No ☐  Describe: _____

_____

Rescue medication if given: _____

Taken to vet? Yes ☐  No ☐  Detail: _____

How long did your dog take to recover? _____

Notes: _____

_____

_____

_____

_____

# *Seizure Log*

| What Happened During the Seizure? | | | |
|---|---|---|---|
| The seizures started with the head | | The seizure started with the limbs | |
| The seizures started on the left / right | | My dog fell down | |
| Stiff body | | Floppy body | |
| Leg paddling | | Shaking | |
| Frothing / drooling | | Chewing movements | |
| Urination | | Defecation | |
| Weakness or twitching in one part of body | | Twitching on one side of face | |
| My dog could see | | My dog could hear | |
| Other: | | Other: | |

| What Happened After the Seizure? | | | |
|---|---|---|---|
| Wobbly | | Weakness in the limbs | |
| Blindness | | Sniffing | |
| Pacing | | Disorientated | |
| Sleepy / tired | | Clingy | |
| Behaviour change: Aggressive / Fearful | | Staring into space / standing in corners | |
| Other: | | Other: | |

| Possible Triggers | | | |
|---|---|---|---|
| Time of day | | Seizures were 'due' (regular interval) | |
| Missed / late medication | | Medication change | |
| Missed sleep | | Missed meal | |
| Exercise | | Temperature (too hot / cold) | |
| Sensory (Loud sounds / flashing lights etc.) | | Specific food. Please note: | |
| Other medication, treatments or supplements. Please note: | | Stressful event. Please describe: | |
| Other: | | Other: | |

Printed in Great Britain
by Amazon